The Ketogenic Diet for Beginners

The Complete Guide to the Keto Diet Offering Clarity to Reset and Heal your Body

Table of Contents

Introduction 1
Keto vs Atkins
Keto vs Paleo

Problems With Modern Diet 15
How Diet Has Changed
Back To Basics
Look At Your Diet

The Good Parts Of The Keto Diet 23

Getting Started With Keto 34
How Low is Low?
First Things First
Macronutrients

The Problems With Keto 49
Side Effects
The Dangers of Keto

Ketosis And How To Reach It 61

Reaching Ketosis
Fuel for the Brain
How to Reach Optimal Ketosis
How to Measure Ketosis

Making Keto Work For Everybody 74

Keto on a Budget
Traveling
Keto While Dining Out
Keto and the Holidays

Is Keto A Good Fit? 93

Exercise 106

Keto and Cardio
Weight Lifting and Keto
Supplementing
Keto and Exercise in Harmony

Keto While Vegan 125

An Overview
Limiting Carbs
Simple Alternatives
Egg Substitutes

Getting Enough Fat
Vegan Protein Sources

FAQ 146
Myths 163
Good Foods 167

What to Eat
Foods to Avoid

Shopping List 184
30-Day Meal Plan 190
Conclusion 205

© Copyright 2018 by _____ - All rights reserved.

The following eBook is reproduced below with the goal of providing information that is as accurate and reliable as possible. Regardless, purchasing this eBook can be seen as consent to the fact that both the publisher and the author of this book are in no way experts on the topics discussed within and that any recommendations or suggestions that are made herein are for entertainment purposes only. Professionals should be consulted as needed prior to undertaking any of the action endorsed herein.

This declaration is deemed fair and valid by both the American Bar Association and the Committee of Publishers Association and is legally binding throughout the United States. Furthermore, the transmission, duplication, or reproduction of any of the following work including specific information will be considered an illegal act irrespective of if it is done electronically or in print. This extends to creating a secondary or tertiary copy of the work or a recorded copy and is only allowed with express written consent from the Publisher. All additional right reserved.

The information in the following pages is broadly considered to be a truthful and accurate account of facts and as such any inattention, use or misuse of the information in question by the reader will render any resulting actions solely under their purview. There are no scenarios in which the publisher or the original author of this work can be in any fashion deemed liable for any hardship or damages that may befall them after undertaking information described herein.

Additionally, the information in the following pages is intended only for informational purposes and should thus be thought of as universal. As befitting its nature, it is presented without assurance regarding its prolonged validity or interim quality. Trademarks that are mentioned are done without written consent and can in no way be considered an endorsement from the trademark holder.

Introduction

The easiest way to explain what the Ketogenic diet is- it is a high-fat, low-carbohydrate, and medium-protein diet. When the diet was started, it was a treatment for refractory epilepsy in children. When followed, it causes the body to burn fat for energy instead of carbs.

The majority of carbohydrates people eat are changed to glucose in the body, which is transported around and helps fuel the body and the brain. However, if the body is not given enough carbohydrates, the liver will start to change fat within the body into fatty acids and ketone bodies. These ketones will then move to the brain to replace glucose. The higher level of ketones in the body is what is helping to reduce the chances of epileptic seizures in children.

Almost half of the kids that were placed on this diet ended up seeing a reduction of seizures and these effects continue even after they returned to their normal diet. With a classic keto diet, you consume about a four to one ratio by weight of combined carbohydrates and protein to fat. This is achieved by removing high-carbohydrate foods such as fruits, sugar, starchy veggies, grains, bread, and pasta. People will also increase their consumption of nuts, butter, and cream that is high in fat.

Most fats that are found in foods are LCTs or long-chain triglycerides. However, MCTs or medium-chain triglycerides are consumed more in a keto diet. Most people who follow a keto diet will consume a lot of coconut oil because it has higher levels of MCTs, or they will use MCT oil and add it to their morning cup of coffee.

Everyone's body and needs are going to be slightly different, but your macros will typically look something like this. 60 to 75 percent of your calories should come from fat, 15 to 30 percent of your calories should come from protein, and 5 to 10 percent of your calories should come from carbs.

After a person has been on a keto diet for a few days, the body will enter what is called ketosis, which we will talk about more in detail later. This is where your body will begin to use up all of your stored fat and the fat you eat for energy.

While this may have been originally used to help people who suffered from epilepsy, people began to see how useful it was to drop a few extra pounds. See, when you eat a lot of carbs, the body retains a lot of fluid so that it is able to store those carbs to use as energy. When a lot of carbs aren't consumed, you end up losing all of those stored fluids.

The biggest reason why people choose to start a diet is to get rid of their stored fats. Keto diet literally targets those areas. While in the beginning, it may seem like it would be hard to stick to because you will have to cut out a lot of different foods, there are many different creative ways to make sure that you won't miss out on some tasty meals. And if you do end up sticking with the diet, you will see that your waistline will start shrinking.

While we're on the subject of foods, there are some products out there that are aimed towards ketogenic dieters. FATBAR is a common one. They create snack bars that contain 200 calories, 16 grams of fat, and four grams of net carbs.

For people who love their morning cup of Joe and may have become used to having a vanilla latte every morning, you can switch it to a bulletproof coffee. This is a regular black coffee with a bit of added butter and MCT oil. It gives you the perfect jump of energy to get your day started.

Before we dive into the specifics of the keto diet, let's look at some differences you may be wondering about.

Keto vs. Atkins

These are the two most popular diets that reduce your carb intake drastically, but let's look at how they compare to each other in terms of results, difficulty, and safety.

The Atkins diet and the keto diet would be neck and neck in a race for the most popular low-carb diets. Both don't just cut back on the bad-for-you carbs such as cookies, donuts, and cupcakes, but they also cut out some veggies and the majority of fruits. They limit carbs enough to make you enter ketosis, which makes the body burn fat for fuel after your glucose stores have been depleted. Ketosis plays a big role in both of these diets, and it also affects how easy it is to stick with them.

Let's quickly go through the Atkins diet. It was introduced in 1972 by Robert Atkins, a cardiologist. The original form of it, which is now called Atkins 20, was made up of four phases. The first phase had the most restrictive rules.

Fats and proteins in Atkins are fair game, but carbs are extremely restrictive to between 20 and 25 grams of net carbs, which are the total carbohydrates minus the dietary fiber. All of these carbs should come from cheese, veggies, seeds, and nuts. This phase lasts until you are about 15 pounds away from your goal weight.

Phase two will bring your carb amount to 25 to 50 grams and you can add in foods like yogurt, cottage cheese, and blueberries. This will last until you are ten pounds away from your goal weight.

In phase three, you will increase your carbs to between 50 and 80 grams of net carbs while you are trying to find the best balance. This means, how many carbs are you able to eat before your weight loss stalls. This part should be done slowly and with a bit of trial and error to figure out how many carbs you can consume with gaining weight.

After you have found that number and managed to maintain it for a month, you will hit phase four. This is lifetime maintenance. This part focuses on keeping up with the habits that you developed during the third phase. You can have up to 100 grams of net carbs per day as long as you don't start gaining weight.

There are a lot of different moving parts when it comes to the Atkins diet. With the keto diet, you have only one way to eat for the complete diet. You will lower your carb intake to around five percent of your daily calorie intake. As a result, you enter ketosis and many people will monitor this by using urine strips or blood tests.

A lot of people still only recommend the keto diet for children with epilepsy because getting rid of complete food groups can drastically change the way you eat, which poses some risk. Some evidence suggests that it can help adults that have epilepsy as well, but there needs to be more research.

If not followed safely and properly, the keto diet can cause an increased risk of kidney stones and possible heart disease, as well as deficiencies in essential minerals and vitamins. In addition to that, until your body has adapted, the buildup of ketones can cause bad breath, mental fatigue, headaches, and nausea.

You will most likely lose weight on both of these diets. In the beginning, it will mainly be water weight. There is a chance with both that the water weight will be regained once you start eating normally again. Studies have found that people who followed the Atkins diet lost 4.6 to 10.3 pounds, though they regained some of that by the end of their second year.

Keto and Atkins don't make you count calories. The important thing is to make sure that you stay under your number of net carbs. Keto does need you to make sure you are hitting the right percentage of calories coming from protein and fat as well.

It depends on each individual person as to which diet is the easiest to follow. It all depends on your habits before you begin the diet. Neither of them is easy.

The main difference between these diets is the amount of protein you can consume. Atkins doesn't put a cap on your protein consumption, but keto does. The other difference is having your body in ketosis during the entire diet. Only the keto diet requires you to stay in ketosis. The Atkins diet slowly lets you reintroduce carbs.

This means that the Atkins diet may be a bit more sustainable in the long run since it is not as restrictive.

Keto vs. Paleo

Paleo is another popular diet people talk about a lot. Let's look at how these two diets compare.

The paleo diet is often called "the caveman diet" and is based on the principles of consuming foods that are available for early humans. One of the theories of the paleo diet is that our modern food systems, processing, and production techniques are harming our health. If you change your eating style to the Paleolithic hunter-gatherer, you will be able to support your own natural biological function and improve your health and digestion. Paleo gets rid of the dairy, processed sugar, legumes, and grains.

The majority of foods that paleo dieters eat are:

- Minimally processed sweetener like raw stevia, coconut sugar, maple syrup, and raw honey.

- Select fats and oils like butter/ghee, tallow, lard, avocado oil, olive oil, and coconut oil.

- Vegetables, except for corn.

- Fruits

- Seeds and nuts

- Eggs

- Fish and meat

For the majority of people who follow paleo, it has less to do with the diet and more for healthier lifestyle practices, the impact on the environment, and total body wellness.

There are distinct differences between paleo and keto but they share some characteristics. They both emphasize whole foods. This means they want you to eat foods that haven't been processed. They both get rid of legumes and grains. They may get rid of these foods for different reasons, but they both discourage them.

They both get rid of added sugars and they add in healthy fats. They are both fairly effective for losing weight.

The big difference between the two is that paleo focuses more on ideology and keto mainly focuses on macronutrients. Paleo wants people to follow the diet for lifestyle changes that help them and the environment. The keto diet doesn't have that type of philosophy. It's just a weight loss plan.

Paleo allows you to eat whole food carbs. Paleo restricts some carb sources. It's not technically a low-carb diet. Paleo also doesn't provide you any specific numbers like macronutrients that you have to follow.

The keto diet will allow you to eat some soy foods and dairy. Keto even tends to encourage the consumption of many different dairy foods like high-fat dairies such as butter, heavy cream, and unsweetened yogurt.

Milk and ice cream are prohibited on keto mainly because they don't have as much fat and are high in carbs. You can also eat soybeans, tempeh, and tofu as long as you are still able to reach you macro allotment. Soy milk though is discouraged.

Paleo does not allow soy and restricts the majority of dairy, grass-fed butter being the exception.

Both diets are okay to follow for health reasons, but the paleo diet does provide healthier options for the majority of people. It gives you more flexibility and it isn't as restrictive as keto.

Now that we've gotten that out of the way, let's dive into the ketogenic diet.

Problems with Modern Diet

Everybody is aware of the fact that obesity is on the rise. In the US, a third of all adults are obese, that's around 78.6 million. But obesity isn't the only problem. It's dangerous to the people. Obesity increases the risk of a large number of unwanted health problems such as stroke, some types of cancer, diabetes, and heart disease. In fact, it is one of the leading causes of preventable death in the United States.

Sadly, with our current modern diet, it shouldn't be surprising that society has a problem. Over the past few decades, the food that we eat and the amount of it have changed. We process our foods more, they are fried up and are placed in helpful to-go packages. They also come in super-sized portions.

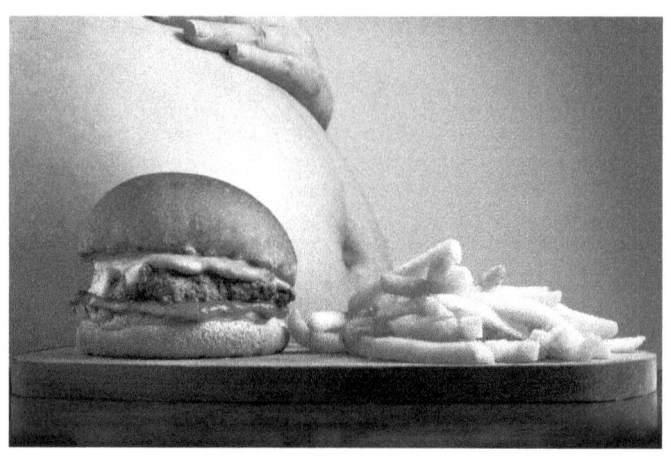

Let's have a deeper look into our modern diet and how it has affected the health of the population.

How Diet Has Changed

In just 30 to 40 years, our diet has drastically changed. Back then, the majority of the foods were fresh and grown locally. People cooked at home. Now, nearly everything that people buy is already processed, even the foods that you cook at home. This comes in the form of trans fats, sugars, colorings, chemicals, additives, and loads of other ingredients that wouldn't have been seen a couple of generations ago.

Additionally, there has been a large increase in sugar consumption over the last few decades. The average American consumes 22 teaspoons of sugar every day, or it makes up 25% of their daily calorie intake. That's an increase of 10% from just ten years ago and a 20% increase since the '70s.

The biggest cause of this is processed fructose, which is typically added to sweeten up desserts, sauces, juices, sodas, and even "healthy" drinks and meals. Kids are also eating more sugar, which is setting them up for a lifetime of poor nutrition and health.

Switching up the fats that we consume has created another problem. For a long time, people have been made to think that coconut oil, animal fats, and other healthy fats could lead to heart problems. People then substituted those fats for processed vegetable oils such as corn and canola. These oils can actually create metabolic changes and hormonal imbalances. Through the years, repeated use of these oils have perpetuated the problem with obesity and more people have turned away from the naturally-occurring, healthy, and important fats that were once used.

With the increased consumption of processed and vegetable oils, we have flooded our bodies with omega-6 fatty

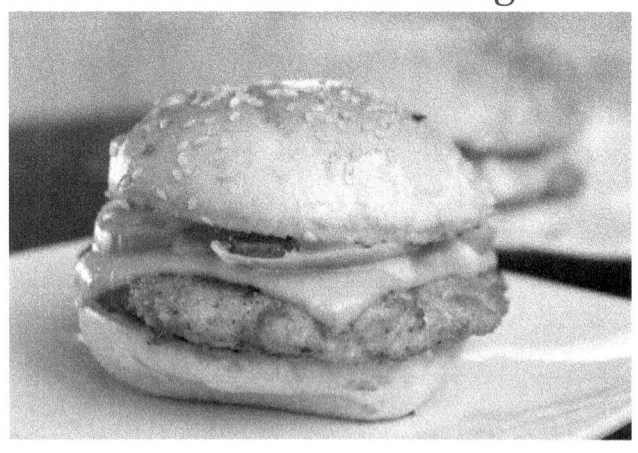

acids. This throws off the balance of fatty acids. When they become imbalanced, it can end up causing some types of cancer, diabetes, arthritis, Alzheimer's, and heart disease. Omega-3 fatty acids, the fats that you find in fish and fish oil, and omega-6 fatty acids need to be balanced. That means you should have one serving for every serving of the other. Today, people tend to eat around twice as many omega-6s than omega-3s.

Convenience foods have also hurt our health. With the fast-paced life of society, more people eat on the go. They grab that fried, fast food that they can easily eat in the car. They grab all of those prepackaged drinks and snacks you find at the gas station. They eat meals that aren't made with natural or fresh foods. It's a trend that may be cheap and easy, but it has done more harm than good.

Back To Basics

The main key to getting our diet back where it should be is to head back to the basics. Centuries ago, cavemen weren't faced with obesity problems. Why? Because they ate foods that came from the earth, fresh fruits, vegetables, unprocessed, untouched foods, and grass-fed meats.

This is how society needs to look at food. People need to add fresh produce to every meal, and instead of staying away from fats, we need to consume good fats for our body to thrive.

The "low fat" phase during the 80s and 90s created a lot of issues for our health. Fats are important for the function of our body. In fact, for the best health, around 50 to 80 percent of our calories need to come from healthy fats. This means beans, eggs, coconut oil, olive oil, seeds, avocado, fish, and nuts. These are all found in nature.

Look At Your Diet

Take a minute to look at your current diet. What type of diet does it resemble? Is it a healthy one like the diet of a prehistoric person? Or is it a disease-riddled modern diet full of fast food? If you chose the latter, you need to make a few changes, both for your own health and your families.

The Good Parts Of The Keto Diet

Now, let me start this chapter with this. In a later chapter, we will be looking at the dangers and side effects that come along with keto diet. I choose to start with the benefits so you would understand why so many people follow the keto diet despite the downsides. So, I want you to take the good and the bad and decide for yourself if it's something you think you can do safely.

Many different things will happen when you follow a ketogenic diet. The following are just a few.

Improvement in Obesity, Metabolic Syndrome and Diabetes

This is the main reason why a lot of people follow a ketogenic diet. In all of the reasons we will look at, plus this reason, a ketogenic diet is perfect for people who suffer from type 1 or type 2 Diabetes. It is also perfect for people who are obese because it is able to help them burn off fat and it spares muscle loss. It is also able to curb a lot of disorders that tend to happen because of obesity. This includes the symptoms and risk factors known as metabolic syndrome.

Improvement in Muscle Gain and Endurance

It has been discovered that BHB helps to promote muscle gain. When you combine this with a lot of anecdotal evidence through the years, a bodybuilder movement has happened with the keto diet and how it can help them gain muscle. Ultra-endurance athletes started to use a keto diet. After an athlete has become fat-adapted, some evidence has suggested that their mental and physical performance has improved.

It Can Help the Eyes

The biggest problem that diabetics could end up facing is macular degeneration. It is common knowledge that high blood sugar can end up hurting a person's eyesight and can lead to a higher risk of cataracts. It shouldn't come as a surprise that when you lower your blood sugar levels, you will also improve your vision and eyes.

Helps Women's Health

In a 2013 review, they found that a keto diet was able to enhance fertility. They also found that PCOS could be treated effectively with a low-carb diet, which was able to reduce or completely eliminate symptoms such as infrequent or prolonged periods, obesity, and acne. Overall, when blood sugar levels are stabilized and low, it will help to equilibrate all of the other hormone levels. This is going to naturally cause a downstream effect of benefits along the metabolic pathways that are connected to insulin such as hunger and energy utilization.

Helps With Gallbladder and Gastrointestinal Health

This means that you will have less bloating and gas, improved digestion, less risk of gallstones, less acid reflux, and heartburn. It's commonly known that sugary foods, nightshades like tomatoes and potatoes, and grain-based foods increase a person's likelihood of heartburn and acid reflux. Therefore, it shouldn't come as a surprise that eating fewer carbs will improve these symptoms and confront the root problems of autoimmune responses, inflammation, and bacterial issues.

A keto diet will also reproducibly and rapidly alter the human gut microbiome. Dr. Eric Westman explains how a large number of problems are removed or reduced because of these microbiome changes. Research has also found that consuming carbs is one of the main causes of gallstones. When you consume enough fats when your carb intake is down, it will help to clear up gallbladders and make things run more smoothly.

Uric Acid Levels Will Stabilize

The biggest culprit of gout and kidney stones are high levels of uric acid, calcium, oxalate, and phosphorus. The main cause of this is typically a combination of consuming things that have a lot of alcohol and purines, unlucky genetics, dehydration, obesity, and sugar consumption. The main caveat is that a ketogenic diet can temporarily raise your uric acid levels, especially if you end up letting yourself become dehydrated. Over time, once you become adapted to the diet and you make sure you consume enough water, your levels will become lower.

Better Energy and Sleep

Once people reach day four or five of the diet, many of them report an increase in energy levels and fewer cravings for carbs. The main reason for this is again stable insulin levels and an energy source that is readily available for the brain and body tissues. It's still a mystery as to why it helps improve sleep. Studies have found that a keto diet improves sleep because it decreases REM and increases slow-wave sleep patterns. The exact reason behind this is unclear. It probably has something to do with the complex biochemical shifts involved in the brain using ketones for energy combined with body burning fat.

Lowered Inflammation

An article in *Nature Medicine* found that it was discovered that the main mechanism behind inflammation that had been believed for decades, a ketogenic diet is an anti-inflammatory diet and it can help with a lot of related issues. Research has discovered that the effects are like connected to "BHB-mediate inhibition of the NLRP3 inflammasome."

Basically, this means that inflammatory disease can be suppressed with BHB, a ketone that is produced when you follow a keto diet. This is how it caused implications concerning arthritis, IBS, acne, eczema, psoriasis, and other inflammatory diseases, and it has prompted a lot more research.

Heart Disease Prevention

A ketogenic diet is able to lower blood pressure and triglyceride level and improve your cholesterol profiles. The reason for this is because of the effects of keeping blood glucose at a low and stable level. While it will likely sound counterintuitive that consuming more fat is going to reduce your triglycerides, it has been discovered that too many carbs are the main reason for high triglyceride levels. When you look at HDL and LDL levels, a keto diet can help to raise your good cholesterol and to lower your bad cholesterol.

Can Fight off Cancer

Dom D'Agostino's lab found that ketone supplementation is able to decrease the viability of tumor cells and prolonged the life of mice that had metastatic cancer. Cancer cell metabolism works abnormally compared to healthy cells. They increase through glucose consumption because of mitochondrial dysfunction and genetic mutations. Some studies have found that unlike healthy tissues, cancer cells can't effectively use ketone bodies for energy. Ketones will also inhibit the viability and proliferation of tumor cells. This doesn't mean a cancer patient should forgo regular treatment. You should still follow your doctor's advice.

Improves the Brain's Focus

The ketogenic diet can help increase memory, clarity, cognition, seizure control, and fewer migraines. The first notable use of the keto diet was in the 1920s at the Mayo Clinic to help children with epilepsy. While the exact reason behind seizure prevention on a keto diet is still unknown, scientists think it's because it causes an increased stability of neurons and upregulation of mitochondrial enzymes and brain mitochondria.

Similar to this, there is a lot of attention given to this diet and its effects on Alzheimer's disease. Researchers have found that there is an increase in cognition and improved memory in adults with problems in these areas, and more research has found improvement in all dementia stages. Ketosis is also able to help fight Parkinson's disease.

For the wider audience of keto diet followers, there are reported side effects of fewer intense and less frequent migraines and better mental focus and clarity. This is likely due to more stable blood sugar and change in brain chemistry that helps cognition and memory too.

Getting Started with Keto

The terms ketogenic and keto can be used interchangeably as you have probably already noticed. The word keto was derived from the fact that when following this type of diet, your body will create small fuel molecules which are called ketones. Your body will use these as an alternative fuel source, which gets used after your body's stored glucose is depleted.

Once you start eating fewer carbs, ketones will be produced. This will remain true as long as your protein intake is kept at a moderate level. Too much protein is able to be switched into sugar just like carbs.

Ketones are created by the liver from the fat stores in your body. The body will then consume these ketones as a fuel source throughout the different areas in your body and the brain. The brain uses way more energy throughout the day than any other part of your body, but it can't run off of fat. The only fuel source that works for the brain is glucose or ketones.

When it comes to following a keto diet, the entire body will switch its fuel supply so that it can run almost completely on fat. This means that your insulin levels are going to drop and you will increase how much fat you burn. Your body will discover that it is easier to access your stored fat and burn them. This is a great byproduct of the keto diet when you are trying to lose some weight, but there are many other less obvious benefits such as mental alertness, lower hunger levels, and steadier energy.

How Low is Low?

The only way that a keto diet will work for you is if you consume very little carbs. The fewer the carbs you eat, the better it will be when it comes to losing weight. This makes the keto diet an extremely strict low-carb diet. The majority of people are only allowed to consume 20 grams or less of net carbs per day. After you have reached your ideal weight, you can then start to increase the carbs you eat. This needs to be done very slowly in order to make sure that you don't gain back the weight you lost.

First Things First

While this is a pretty effective weight loss diet, there is a right and a wrong way to do it. You need to make sure that you start off the right way in order to ensure that you get the best and fastest results.

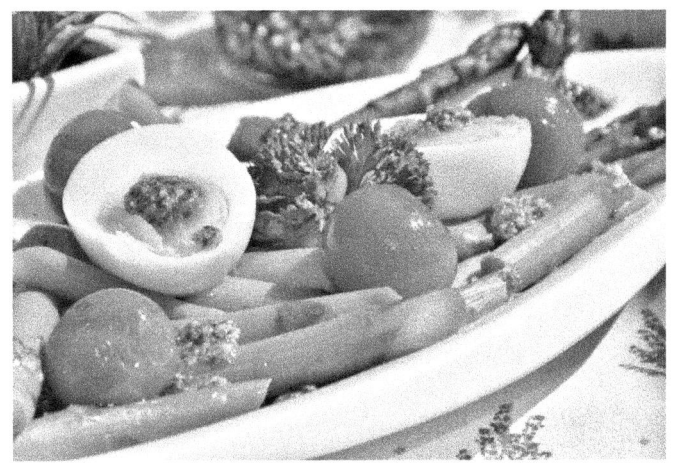

In theory, a ketogenic diet is pretty simple. You eat low amounts of carbs and high amounts of fat. But in practice, it's a bit more complicated. You need to know what you can and cannot eat. In a later chapter, you will find a more complete list of the things that you can and can't eat, but let's have a look at a basic list of these foods.

- Heavy fats such as olive oil, bacon fat, tallow, lard, ghee, butter, and coconut oil.

- Meats and that include organ meats as well.

- Eggs
- Seafood and fish.
- Non-starchy vegetables. You will definitely want leafy greens.
- Some berries, like blueberries, strawberries, and raspberries.

This means that a typical day could look like:

- Breakfast: bacon and eggs.
- Lunch: chicken salad with a cup of bone broth.
- Dinner: steak with a side of veggies and a ketogenic dessert.

There are some people who will eat a snack in between their meals. There isn't any need for a snack unless you need a little energy boost or are feeling a bit hungry. Some good snack ideas are meat sticks, celery sticks, nuts, broth, and cheese sticks. You have to keep an eye on your snacks though, they will add to your complete macro count.

You can also easily personalize the keto diet. You have the power to experiment with things to see what is going to work best for you. There are some people who discover that they need to eat more fats while other people are able to eat a lot fewer carbs. Some people even use intermittent fasting.

The majority of those people who choose to follow intermittent fasting will skip breakfast and eat their first meal at one. This will raise their ketosis. There are a lot of people who find that they naturally fall into intermittent fasting because they don't feel as hungry. And that's fine too.

Macronutrients

Macros have already been mentioned several times in this book and you are probably ready to learn more about them. Macro is a short-term for macronutrients when you are talking about a ketogenic diet.

Macros are the different parts of the food that you eat which provides you with energy and fuel. The three macros are protein, fat, and carbohydrates. These are the areas where all of your dietary calories are going to come from. This is probably the biggest thing that you really need to learn in order to make sure that you are successful with the keto diet. You need to make sure that they stay in the right balance in order to ensure that you remain in ketosis.

Carbohydrates are the only macro that you don't have to consume in order to survive. There are essential amino acids and fatty acids which are the building blocks of proteins and fats, but there aren't any essential carbohydrates.

Carbs are made up of two things, starches and sugars. Fiber is viewed as a carb, but with a keto diet, it isn't counted towards a total carb intake. The reason fiber isn't counted is that the body doesn't really digest fiber, so it doesn't have much of an effect on your blood sugar.

This means, when you pick up something and read its nutritional label, the first thing that you need to look at is the total carbs. Then have a look at the dietary fiber. After that, you will need to subtract the amount of fiber content from the total carb amount. This is going to give you what is known as net carb content.

It looks like this:

Total carbs – fiber = net carbs

This makes sure that the only carbs that are counted are the starches and the sugars in each of the carbohydrates. When you have to figure out the macros in a meal, you will only have to look at the net carbs and you don't have to look at the complete carbs. Now, there are some foods that don't contain any dietary fiber, and in that case, you would use the complete carb amount.

In order to make sure that you succeed, you will need to figure out the foods that are naturally low in carbs and the ones that are not. Not all of these foods sources will be obvious. Everybody knows potatoes are high in carbs, they are starchy, but did you realize that bananas are also high in carbs?

Before we get into the nitty gritty of figuring out your macro numbers, a basic rule of them is that you shouldn't consume more than 20 grams of net carbs every day.

It's crucial that you consume enough protein because it is important for the body. It helps to preserve your lean muscle mass, it's an energy source when there aren't any carbs, it creates enzymes and hormones, it helps the immune function, repairs tissue, and helps it grow. The biological process requires protein. Proteins are the building blocks for a healthy body.

When you eat proteins, your body will break them down into amino acids. Nine of the amino acids that protein produces are cannot be produced by the body alone. This is the reason why these essential amino acids must come from the foods you eat. These nine amino acids are valine, tryptophan, threonine, phenylalanine, methionine, lysine, leucine, isoleucine, and histidine. When you have protein deficiency or a deficiency in any of these amino acids, it can end up causing malnutrition, kwashiorkor, or a whole host of other health problems.

When you follow a ketogenic diet, it's imperative that you make sure that you eat enough protein in order to preserve your lean body mass. The amount that you consume will greatly depend on how much lean body mass you currently have. Here is a guideline.

- .7 to .8 grams of protein per pound of muscle to help preserve your muscle mass.

- .8 to 1.2 grams of protein per pound of muscle to help you increase your muscle mass.

Your goal should never be to lose body mass. You should only want to preserve or gain it. There are a lot of people that are focused on losing weight, but there are times that losing weight will cause you to lose muscle along with fat. Your goal should be to lose fat and save your muscle. This plays an important role in making sure that you keep a good metabolism.

The main thing you need to remember is that you shouldn't go overly crazy when eating protein on a ketogenic diet. Too much protein could end up stressing your kidneys too much and it could affect your level of ketosis. As long as you keep your macros in the appropriate range, all should be okay.

Here is a great example to go by.

Let's assume that you weigh 160 pounds and you have 30 percent body fat. This means you have around 48 pounds of body fat. Then you can subtract your body fat from your total weight. This will give you your lean body mass. For this example, it would be 112 pounds.

To figure out how much protein you should consume, you have to take the lean body mass number and multiply by the ratio from earlier. For this example, you would have to consume 89.6 grams of protein each day to preserve your muscle mass. The computation looks like this.

112 pounds muscle x .8 grams protein = 89.6 grams

The macro we need to go over is fat. Fat needs to be consumed in adequate amounts in order for your body to maintain cell membranes, provide protective cushioning for organs, absorb certain vitamins, development, growth, and energy. With the keto diet, fats also help you to stay full.

In the body, dietary fat is broken into glycerol and fatty acids. The body isn't able to synthesize two types of fatty acids, so you have to make sure that you consume them in your regular diet. These include linoleic acid and linolenic acid.

These fats are sating, so it's perfect for people looking to fight off hunger pangs. Now you have to figure out how much fat you need to eat. If your carbs are at a minimum, you've figured out how much protein you need to eat, and then the rest of your dietary needs have to be met with fat.

To maintain weight, you will eat enough calories from fat to support your regular expenditure. If you want to burn fat, then you will have to eat in a deficit.

Now, I have given you a lot of information to help you figure out your macros. However, there is a lot easier way to figure this out. There are a lot of online calculators to figure out these numbers without getting a headache. If you want to use an online calculator, check out the website Ketogains. They have one that works great.

Now, if you want to see how figuring it out on your own will work, let's continue with the 160-pound example from earlier. Let's say this person is a female, stands 5'4", in her late 20s, and has a desk job. She's mainly sedentary.

Plugging in her info into a calculator:

The base metabolic rate would be 1467 kcal.

Daily energy expenditure would be 1614 kcal.

She would need to eat around 90 grams of protein, 20 grams of net carbs, and 86 grams of fat. Her intake is made up of 72 percent fat, 23 percent protein, and 5 percent carbs.

Now you know what macros are and how to figure out your numbers. You are well on your way to getting started with a ketogenic diet.

The Problems With Keto

While for the most part, the ketogenic diet is a safe and effective diet, it does come with some dangers and sides effects. Before we go into the dangers of keto, let's look at the most common side effects that you could end up experiencing once your body enters ketosis.

Side Effects

Not all of the side effects of the ketogenic diet are bad, but there are going to be some unpleasant ones that you may experience.

1. Very little energy.

This is a very common problem when your body is starting to adjust to your new source of energy. Luckily, after your body has adjusted to using fat as energy, your energy will go up.

2. You A1C levels could improve.

If you are diabetic, the better blood sugar control could help to control your A1C and it might even reduce your need for insulin. That doesn't mean you should go off your meds though. The only caveat is that it does also increase your risk of diabetic ketoacidosis, which is life-threatening. This is more common for people with type 1 diabetes, but if you have type 2, you should still talk to your doctor first.

3. You won't have as much brain fog.

It is a well-known fact that carbs, especially the refined kinds like white pasta, white bread, and sugar will end up causing your blood sugar to spike and then dip. So it's very easy to see why when you eat fewer carbs, you will be able to keep your blood sugar levels steady. For healthy people, this means that they will keep a steady energy level, less brain fog, and fewer sugar cravings.

4. You may notice that your skin clears up.

If you have been bothered by pimples, you could find that the keto diet could clear them up. This is especially true if you used to be a sugar addict. Empty carbs are the worst thing for acne because they trigger inflammation. Some studies have found that curbing your carb intake could fix those types of problems.

5. You will have increased thirst.

You shouldn't worry if you start to notice that you feel more parched when you start your keto diet. Your body is going to be excreting a lot more water and this will make you thirsty. The important thing is to remember that you drink plenty of water. There is no exact amount that you have to drink, but you should make sure that you drink enough water to turn your urine clear to pale yellow.

6. You may notice that you are feeling less hungry.

Most diets are associated with fighting off cravings and feeling hungry. That's not necessarily the case with the keto diet. There are a lot of people who report less hunger and a diminished need for eating. Researchers aren't completely sure why this happens, but it's believed that low carb diets suppress the hormone ghrelin which controls hunger.

7. Your weight will likely drop quickly, but you may notice that some come back.

The reason the ketogenic diet became so popular is that of its initial quick slim down. The reason for this is because your body will release quite a bit of water when you switch to using fat as energy. The scales will likely show that you have lost a few pounds and you could even look leaner.

That first drop in weight that you notice is likely going to be just water weight. This doesn't mean that you've not burned off fat. The problem comes with the fact that while studies have discovered that you will lose weight, they have yet to figure out if it can be sustained. Most people will find that this type of strict diet is hard to stick to. If you do veer off of your diet, you could find that you gain some of the weight back.

8. You can end up feeling sick and tired.

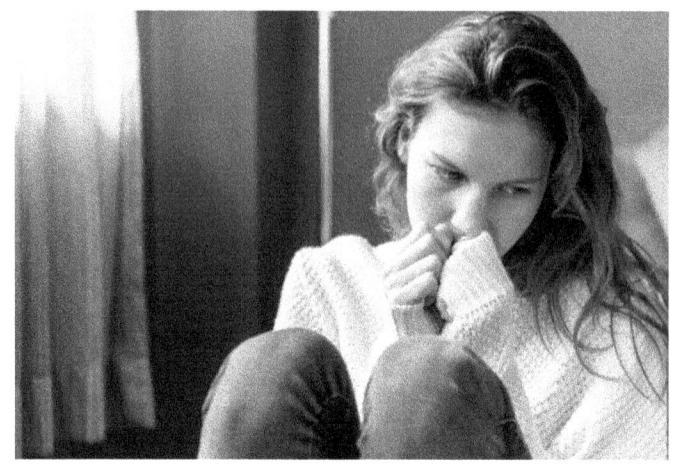

The keto flu is completely real. When you cut your carbs and reach ketosis, it will bring about a number of uncomfortable symptoms such as diarrhea, nausea, muscle aches, fatigue, and headaches. These side effects are caused by the body transitioning into using fat as its main energy source instead of carbs. Once your body has adapted to this fuel source in about a week or two, you will notice that you feel a lot better.

The Dangers of Keto

Now, we've talked through some of the side effects that you could experience until your body gets used in using fat as a fuel source. The negative side effects will go away. The following things that could happen when following a keto diet may not. These are all rare things and typically will only happen if you don't eat healthily and follow your macros, but it could end up happening. It's important to know them so that you can avoid them.

1. Cardiac Issues

Losing some heart muscle isn't the only heart-associated risk that could come along with the keto diet. If you are already on medication for high blood pressure and you are on the keto diet, you could end up with abnormally low blood pressure results. If you already have a heart condition, talk to your doctor before you start a keto diet.

2. Muscle Loss

The longer you allow your body to stay in ketosis, the more fat it is going to burn. But you could cause your body to start burning off muscle tissue too. While consuming enough protein does wonders for building up muscle, your muscles can also use carbs for their formation and maintenance. Without consuming carbs, your body could possibly start breaking down its own muscles.

3. Kidney Damage and Stones

If you do let yourself get dehydrated and you don't take control of it quickly, it could end up causing acute kidney injury. But this isn't the only way that it could cause damage to your kidneys. Too much protein can end up creating high nitrogen levels which will cause the pressure in your kidneys to increase. This may end up creating kidney stones that can end up hurting your kidney cells.

4. Dehydration

This is a very common thing for people who are just starting the keto diet because ketosis will cause your body to flush out excess water. In order to prevent dehydration, you should try to aim for 2.5 liters of water every day. You need to start drinking this much water as soon as you start a ketogenic diet. You do not need to wait until you start noticing the side effects of dehydration.

5. Decreased Serum Sodium

Most Americans will consume too much salt, but for a person that is following a ketogenic diet, they can sometimes struggle to consume enough. Low sodium levels can end up causing confusion, leg cramps, decreased energy, and vomiting. Make sure that all of your meals have salt added to them. Sea salt is the best choice because it also contains trace minerals.

6. Loss of Electrolytes

When you hit ketosis, your body will start to dump stores of glycogen which is found in your muscles and fat that carries extra weight. This will make you use the bathroom more and will lead to electrolyte loss. Electrolytes are important for proper cardiac function and normal heartbeats. This could cause a cardiac arrhythmia. Try to get more electrolytes through natural sources or through OTC supplements.

7. Bowel Changes and Constipation

Besides not getting their nutrients, eliminating veggies and fruits causes other problems as well. They are fiber-rich foods that help keep you regular. Without those foods, you may find that you start having bowel changes which include difficulty in bowel movements and possible constipation.

You will need to make sure you load up on fiber-rich, low-carb foods like cabbage, asparagus, and broccoli, as well as more fats like ghee and coconut oil.

8. Nutritional Deficiencies

A high-fat, low-carb diet will limit the kinds of foods that you are able to eat and complete food groups will be eliminated. Whole grains, beans, and legumes are all out, and so are a lot of vegetables and fruits. Most of the foods carry nutrients, vitamins, and minerals that you aren't able to get anywhere else. Without those foods, you could end up experiencing nutritional deficiencies.

Keto isn't good for a long-term diet because it's not balanced. Diets that are devoid of veggies and fruits will cause long-term micronutrient deficiencies that will come along with other consequences. It's great for short-term fat loss, but it is best under the supervision of a medical professional.

9. Low Blood Sugar

For the most part, once you have reached ketosis, you will notice more stable and lower blood sugar levels. That's why low-carb diets are effective at controlling type 2 diabetes. Carb monitoring has been used for a while now as a way to control blood sugar. But one study has found that low-carb diets aren't better for long-term control than any other diet.

There is some anecdotal evidence that says people with type 2 diabetes were able to stop taking their medicine because they were about to stabilize their blood sugar. But that is in no way recommended and people with diabetes must talk to their doctor first.

Those first few days while the body is adapting to the changes, your body is in a constant struggle. You will need to ease your way into the diet if you have diabetes. Slowly cut back on your carbs, otherwise, you could cause your blood sugar to drop too much.

Ketosis and How to Reach It

We've talked about ketosis a lot. We've even talked about what it does to the body. There is still a lot about ketosis that you have yet to learn, like how to get into it and what it means to your health. Let's look even further into what it is. The important thing to know is that ketosis is a natural state that your body will enter when it is being fueled by fat. This can happen if a person fasts or if they follow a very strict low-carb diet.

There are many different benefits for ketosis like performance, health, and weight loss. But like what we talked in the last chapter, it also comes along with some unpleasant side effects. For people who have type 1 diabetes and certain other disease types, too many ketones in their body can end up becoming dangerous.

Once your body enters ketosis, it will start to produce ketones. Ketones are small fuel molecules and the body will use them as an alternative source of energy once your glucose stores have been depleted. The liver will change your fat into ketones that are then sent into the blood. The body will then use the ketones just like it used glucose. Ketones can also fuel the brain.

Reaching Ketosis

There are two ways for your body to reach ketosis: A Ketogenic diet or fasting. Under either one of these circumstances, once the body's limited amount of glucose has been depleted, the body will switch its source for fuel to fat. The fat-storing hormone, insulin, will become low, and the body's fat burning will be increased. This means that your body has easy access to your fats stores and can get rid of them.

You are considered to be in ketosis once your body produces enough ketones to make a significant level in the blood, usually more than .5mm. The quickest way for this to happen is through fasting, but it isn't something you can do forever. That is why people turn to a keto diet because it can be eaten for an indefinite amount of time.

Fuel for the Brain

A lot of people think you have to have carbs to fuel your brain. The brain will happily burn carbs when you consume them, but when carbs aren't available it will happily eat ketones.

This is necessary for basic survival. Since the body is only able to store carbs for a day or two, the brain would end up shutting down after a few days with no food. Alternatively, it would need to quickly convert muscle protein into glucose, which isn't very efficient just in order to keep working. That would mean we could waste away very quickly. If this was the way the body worked, then the human race wouldn't have been able to survive before 24/7 food became available.

The body has evolved to work smarter than that. Normally, the body will have fat stores that will last so that a person can survive for several weeks without food. Ketosis is the process that happens to make sure that the brain is able to run on those fat stores.

How to Reach Optimal Ketosis

This is what everybody on a ketogenic diet wants. When you reach optimal ketosis, your body will burn fat at the most optimal speed. To reach this optimal ketosis, you have to follow the low-carb, high-fat diet as laid out above, keeping your macros in the optimal range. There isn't any trick to help you reach this optimal level. There are some things you can do.

Here are the different ketone levels you could have.

- Below 0.5 means that you are not in ketosis.

- Between 0.5 and 1.5 is a light level of nutritional ketosis. You will be losing weight, but it won't be optimal.

- Around 1.5 to 3 is what is considered optimal ketosis and is best for maximum weight loss.

- Levels over 3 aren't needed. High levels aren't going to help you one way or the other and could end up harming you because it could mean that you aren't getting enough food.

There are a lot of people who believe that they are consuming a strict keto diet but end up being surprised when they measure their blood ketone levels. When measured, they end up being around 0.2 or 0.5, which isn't at that sweet spot.

The trick to get past this plateau is that you not only have to avoid the obvious carb sources but making sure your protein intake doesn't get higher than your fat intake. I know I said protein won't affect your glucose levels as easily as carbs do, but if you consume too many, especially if you eat more than fat, it will affect your glucose. This will compromise your optimal ketosis.

The secret to working around this problem is to increase your intake of fat. You can do this by adding a big dollop of herbed butter to your steak. This could keep you from eating as much or going back for seconds.

Having a glass of bulletproof coffee can also help to stave off hunger and prevents you from eating as much protein. This is as simple as adding a tablespoon of butter and a tablespoon of coconut oil to your coffee in the morning.

The more fats you eat, the fuller you will feel. This will make sure that you don't eat too much protein and you will eat fewer carbohydrates. This should help you to reach optimal ketosis.

How to Measure Ketosis

There are a few ways to figure out whether or not you have reached ketosis. The first way is measuring ketones in your blood. This requires purchasing a meter and will require a prick on the finger.

There are quite a few reasonably priced gadgets out there for this, and it only takes a few seconds to find out what your blood ketone level is. Most people don't go to this extreme to find out what their ketone level is, but it is the most accurate and effective.

You should measure your blood ketones first thing in the morning and on a fasted stomach. You can follow the levels that I listed earlier in this chapter to figure out if you are in ketosis.

These meters measure the amount of BHB that you have in your blood. This is the main ketone that will be present when in ketosis. The main downside of using this method is the fact that you have to draw blood.

Finding a test kit will cost around $30 to $40, and could cost an extra $5 for every test. This is the reason why those who choose to test this way will only perform one test every week or every other week.

All right, so if you don't want to go to the expense of getting a blood ketone meter, we've got six other options to figure out whether or not you are in ketosis.

1. Bad breath

This doesn't sound pleasant but people will often say they have bad breath when they hit ketosis. This is a fairly common side effect. People will often say that their breath becomes fruitier.

The reason for this is the elevated ketone levels. The main culprit is the ketone acetone that the body excretes through your breath and urine. While you may not like the idea of having bad breath, it is a great way to know you're in ketosis. A lot of people will brush their teeth more often or chew sugar-free gum.

2. Ketones in urine and breath

If you don't want to prick your finger, you can measure blood ketones with a breath analyzer. This will monitor for acetone which is one of the three ketones that will be present in your blood once you reach ketosis.

This will let you know when your ketone levels have hit ketosis level because acetone will only leave the body once you reach nutritional ketosis. These breath analyzers are fairly accurate, though not as accurate as a blood monitor.

Another way to check for ketosis is to check for ketones in the urine every day using special indicator strips. This is a quick and cheap method to use to assess what your ketone levels are every day. These aren't the most reliable methods though.

3. Better energy and focus

A lot of people will sometimes report feeling sick, tired, or have brain fog once they first start a keto diet. This is the keto flu, but people who follow this long-term will report better energy and increased focus. Your body has to take the time to adapt to the new diet. Once you hit ketosis, your brain will start burning ketones for energy and this could take a week or so to start happening.

Ketones are a more potent fuel source for the brain as opposed to carbs. This means that it will improve your mental clarity and brain function.

4. Short-term performance decrease

Just like with number three, the fatigue can cause a decrease in exercise performance. This is due to the reduction in your muscle glycogen stores, which is what typically provides you with the fuel you need for high-intensity exercises. After a week or so your performance levels should return to normal.

5. Digestive issues

With the major changes to the foods you eat, you will probably experience diarrhea or constipation in the beginning. This lets you know that you are reaching ketosis. After your transition period, these issues should go away.

6. Insomnia

One of the biggest issues a keto dieter will have is insomnia especially when they first start. When a person's carbs are drastically reduced, it can cause sleeping issues. However, this too shall pass.

There are a lot of different signs and symptoms that will let you know if you are in ketosis and if you are doing things correctly. Ultimately, if you follow the rules for a keto diet and you keep yourself consistent, your body will be in some form of ketosis.

If you want to know absolutely for certain whether or not you are in ketosis, the only way to do that is with a blood ketone monitor.

Making Keto Work For Everybody

Most people will stay away from diets if they think they are too hard to put into their lives. The great thing about the keto diet is, it isn't that hard to implement and it shouldn't interfere with your life in any way. To help everyone feel like they can follow a keto diet, this chapter will look at eating on a budget, eating out, eating during the holiday, and even more.

Keto on a Budget

Many people assume that eating keto will be expensive, but it really isn't. Your fat intake is going to be upped. Fats help make you feel fuller than carbs will. This means that you can go longer between meals. Not eating snacks all the time will help you save money too.

Since protein levels aren't really going to change, you aren't going to be faced with having to buy expensive meats. Here are some money-saving tips.

- Keep things simple. Your meals don't have to be difficult and have many different parts. The fewer ingredients you use, the less money you are going to spend. If you make a simple omelet and drink water, it is going to cost you about $3.50. A Big Mac will cost you $5.

- You get a better deal if you buy a whole chicken and cut it up yourself. Keep the bones too. You can use it to make broth.

- Buy fresh vegetables when they are in season. The rest of the year, you can purchase frozen.

- Watch for sales at your grocery store. Stock up on these items especially if you use a lot of them.

It also helps if you can plan out your meal in advance and make a shopping list. This will ensure you stay organized. You will just buy what you need. Planning your shopping list is the best way to stop all unnecessary spending and impulse buying.

While shopping, here are some things you can do to save money.

- Purchase regular cheese. There is no reason to purchase the expensive specialty cheeses. Buy in bulk if you can, and never purchase pre-shredded. Find a block of cheese and shred it yourself.

- Just like cheese, buy simple meats and avoid specialty ones. Cooked meats make a fast meal but choose the less exotic types.

- Don't buy the bags of coleslaw. Buy a head of cabbage and shred it yourself. It will last longer and you will get more meals out of it.

- Don't worry about finding kale. Find other leafy greens that are cheaper and just as nutritious.

- Only buy avocados when they are in season.

- Stop buying nuts because these get expensive, especially macadamias.

- Get an almond meal instead of almond flour. It is cheaper and works as well as almond flour in recipes. You could also grind your own almonds.

- Buy frozen or canned fish instead of fresh, especially when talking about salmon.

Get the best quality foods that you can afford. Just because everyone says you need to eat organic doesn't mean you absolutely have to. If you can't afford something, then don't get it. The important thing is that you make your meals at home from scratch. They will be healthier even if they aren't organic.

When choosing meats, go with a cheaper cut and make sure you look for bargains or reduced meats.

You need to cook all of your meals at home. This is cheaper and healthier than eating out. Go with easy recipes and avoid all the fancy keto recipes.

Traveling

The most important part of any diet is maintaining it when you aren't at home. The key to making sure you maintain your diet is planning. The following will help you maintain your diet while you are traveling.

- Know your macros

Before taking a vacation, you need to know what your macros are. Make sure you have them memorized or have a keto app on your phone that helps track your macros.

- Food options

You must think about the foods you can take. Non-perishable foods are the best options. Canned salmon, tuna, chicken, and beef jerky are all great options. Canned shakes and olives are also great to take with you. All of your snacks like string cheese, pepperoni, and dried nuts are also great. If you like eating eggs, hard boil them to take them along.

When talking about foods that need refrigeration, if you aren't traveling too far from home, you should purchase any perishables when you have arrived. This is where it is important to have a refrigerator at the place you are staying.

Once you arrive, go to the store and buy your cheese and meats. One other option is making your meals ahead of time and freezing them before a trip. Pack them in a cooler and put them in the freezer once you arrive. Every morning, set the meals for that day in the refrigerator to thaw.

- Travel evaluation

You need to know how long your trip is going to take. If it is just overnight, it is going to be fairly easy to prepare. You just need a few frozen meals, a microwave, and a cooler. If your trip is going to be all week, it does change things and create complications. You have to know what you are going to be up against.

Once you have your location and length of your trip, begin to look at resources that will be available to you when you get there.

It is good to book a place that has a kitchen in it like an Airbnb. If you are staying at a hotel, find a room at an extended-stay hotel. These places have better cooking equipment than normal motels and hotels. This increases your flexibility when prepping meals. It would be great if you could find a place that has a full-size refrigerator and freezer. Staying with family and friends is good since you would have access to a full kitchen.

How you get to your destination is important too. If you are driving, you have more flexibility than traveling by plane. TSA restrictions might prevent you from bringing specific foods with you because they need to be repacked and weigh less than three ounces.

- Restaurants

Many restaurants and fast food places offer low carb options now. If you want a burger, just ask them to wrap it in a lettuce leaf or just leave off the bun. Choosing meats like steak and fish will keep you on your low-carb diet. Never order fries or potatoes. Stay away from rice and beans. Instead, order roasted vegetables, asparagus, and salads. If there is a Chipotle near you, you can get a bowl without bean or rice and fill it with guacamole, sour cream, cheese, and meat.

Traveling doesn't mean you have to stop your diet. There are many ways to work around this. It really isn't that hard if you plan ahead.

Keto While Dining Out

Have you been asked out by friends? Are you afraid to go? You don't have to be. You can eat delicious foods no matter where you go.

- Avoid starches

Stay away from bread. Say no to pasta. Pass on the potatoes. Bounce the rice. Never put temptations on your plate. Make sure you order meals without starchy sides.

When ordering an entrée, most places let you substitute the starchy sides for more vegetables or a salad. When you order a sandwich or burger, ask for it to be wrapped in lettuce instead. If they won't make any changes, just don't order it.

When you get your plate and it has a starch on it, look at the options. If you can leave it there and not eat it, go for it. If you can't handle the temptation, ask the server to replace it to get rid of the starch. If the restaurant is casual, you can take care of things by just throwing it away.

- Be careful with condiments and sauces

Sauces like Bearnaise sauce contain mostly fats. Ketchup contains many carbs. Gravies might end up going either way. If you aren't sure about a particular sauce, ask what's in it and stay away if it has sugar or flour in it. You could also ask if they would place the sauce on the side so you could choose whether or not to eat it.

- Add good fats

Restaurant meals are usually low in fats. This makes it hard for us to feel full when not eating carbs. You can change this in many different ways. Ask for extra butter and put it on your vegetables or meats. Choose a vinegar and olive oil based dressing for your salad. Many restaurants serve cheap vegetable oils that are full of Omega 6 fatty acids instead of olive oil. An advanced keto dieter will carry a small bottle of olive oil with them.

- Choose drinks wisely

The best choices would be sparkling water, unsweetened tea, coffee, and water. If you want an alcoholic beverage, choose a dry wine, champagne, or spirits, either straight or with club soda.

- Dessert

If you aren't hungry, have a cup of coffee to finish off your meal. If you still feel a bit hungry, see if they have a cheese plate or some berries and whipped cream.

- Buffets

This is when things can get tricky. Set ground rules before you leave the table. Stay away from all grains and starches and aim for proteins, vegetables, and fats. Find the smallest plate and go back for more if the first plate doesn't fill you up. Be sure you take your time eating. Talk with friends and sip on your drink.

Keto and the Holidays

Holidays are always going to happen. These are the hardest times of the year to stay on any diet. This is the time to sit on the couch, eat too much, and watch too much television. This is fine, but this doesn't mean you have to stop doing keto. It is during these times when you need to reevaluate yourself and check on your keto lifestyle. Take a look at the progress you've made already and learn how to move past these anxiety-inducing moments. Here's how.

1. Keep a Keto Positive Mind

What does it mean to have a keto positive mind? Look at it like the Commandments of the Low Carb Followers. Thou shalt not drool over thy neighbor's turkey sandwich, thou shalt not make friends feel bad for having fries, thou shalt not gloat, and so on. You, you are doing keto, but you are also a compassionate and an awesome person too. Keep yourself composed and stay on keto.

2. Knowledge is Power

There are tons of apps out there that you can download for free that lets you know what is in the food you are about to eat. This means, if you see some cheese making its rounds at a party, you don't have to feel bad for tasting it. The trick to succeeding during the holidays is knowing what to say yes to and by making smart decisions. MyFitnessPal is a great choice to keep track of meals and figuring out what is in your food.

3. Create Clear Goals

The best way to make sure that you stay on track is to come up with clear goals. Everybody's keto lifestyle is a little bit different. The rules you come up will need to be based on what your goals are, which will end up determining your actions. If you're looking to drop excess fat, that's going to look different than somebody that is trying maintain or gain. A keto-warrior could have a five-point backup plan. The best goals are your own goals.

4. Plan to Fail

What does it mean to plan to fail? This means you set the bar so high that even if you don't reach your goal, you still have done better than your expectations. This is the best win-win situation. It's also very easy to do. If you know desserts are your weakness, make your own keto cheesecake and take it to the party. Now you can have your cake and eat it too.

5. Never Engage in a Debate

When you get into the keto lifestyle, you might find it tempting to try to convert others to your way of life. But it's important to understand that not everybody wants to take that step, especially when it comes to the holidays. Your aunt may not understand the reason why you have bacon for every meal of the day and nor does she want to. The important thing is to make sure you are taking the steps you need to in order to stay on track. You don't have to look out for the entire family.

6. Plan Things Away from the Couch or Table

One easy way to stay keto is to change how you see everything. Instead of waiting for people to invite you to a party, where you end up anxious about what foods they will have, make the plans yourself. Invite your family and friends on a trip, a walk around town, or to see a show. There are a lot of free events around the holidays and everybody will feel happier with some exercise.

7. Be Gracious and Have an Escape

This brings us to another point, the holidays tend to be hard for everybody. There's lots of traveling, lots of families and everybody has to make sacrifices. That could mean you have to chock down your mom's overseasoned meatloaf, but do it with a smile on your face because it's the holidays. A small sacrifice isn't going to be a big deal when you look at the grander scheme of things. You could also try to keep from visiting around mealtimes.

8. Cheating is Fine, Just Set Some Rules

A huge taboo for keto land is cheating. When somebody breaks the rules and eats something that they regret, they end up sitting around lambasting their self for weeks on end. Stop it. You are in charge of the rules and you can change those rules. If you have a round of fries, it doesn't mean you have screwed everything up. Don't take these slips so hard and it will be easier to get back on track.

9. Remain Calm

The holidays only come around once every year, but you have keto for the rest of your life. If you have to take a few weeks off and enjoy all the great festivities, go ahead. If you feel like you need to up your gym time to make up for some carb eating, do it. If you are a keto warrior, then keto on. Nobody is going to judge you for trying to do your best during the craziest time of year. Don't kill yourself over having too many cookies, or that cup of apple cider. Just get back on track and everything is going to be fine.

10.   Say Thank You

You are going to be offered all sorts of things. It's what happens during the holidays. The best thing to do is say thank you, accept it, and continue to talk. Odds are, they won't even notice that you didn't eat their fudge. If you tell them no, it might upset them. Repeat after me, "Awesome, thank you," take it and smile.

Is Keto A Good Fit?

The keto diet gets a lot of praises for being a wonderful weight loss plan. This high-fat, low-carb life might not be right for you.

You might have read some articles about this diet already. It might sound just like any other fad diet that won't last. Truth is, this diet has been around for over 100 years. This diet has many health benefits. Research has shown us this diet can help lose weight, prevent obesity, improve alertness and cognition, improve metabolic and cardiovascular conditions, and treat epilepsy.

This happens when you get into ketosis. Our bodies go through various phases of hormonal and metabolic adaptations so it learns how to use the new source of energy it is getting from fat.

When our bodies don't have glucose available for fuel, these fatty acids will get turned into ketones that go across the blood-brain barrier that will give the heart, muscles, and brain more energy. It minimizes all the excess fat that has been stored in our bodies.

Just like any diet, there are some safety problems that you have to keep in mind. The keto diet isn't right for every person. Here are some situations where the keto diet might be dangerous and you should avoid it.

Nursing or Pregnant

There haven't been many studies done to figure out all the side effects of the keto diet on pregnant women. Studies have shown some of the side effects may include constipation, anemia, inadequate growth in children, hormonal changes, nutrient deficiency, dehydration, and weight loss.

Prolonged ketosis when pregnant can cause developmental problems with the baby that can affect how well their brains develop and increase the risk of birth defects such as spina bifida.

Because of all the risk of possible harm to the baby, doctors do not recommend this diet to pregnant women.

Just like with pregnant women, there haven't been many studies done about the keto diet and nursing women. Many women who are either nursing or pregnant need more protein and fiber than women who are not pregnant or nursing. The increased fiber helps to support fetal development and growth. It helps improve the mom's digestion and gives both mom and the baby the minerals and vitamins they need.

Because we don't really know the exact results of a keto diet on moms who are nursing, it is best to adopt a moderate carb intake that keeps both mom and the baby safe.

Medicines That Could Cause Hypoglycemia

These medicines can cause hypoglycemia.

- Sulphonylureas like glipizide, tolbutamide, gliclazide, glimepiride, and glibenclamide
- Glinides like repaglinide or nateglinide
- Insulin

These medicines were designed to help the body increase insulin levels. This, in turn, lowers blood sugar.

If you follow a keto diet while taking these medications, it might cause you to develop hypoglycemia. It is very important to talk to your doctor so you can work together to prevent the risk of developing hypoglycemia before you start a keto diet.

Testing your blood sugar allows you to spot and possibly avoid developing hypoglycemia. You are going to have to test more often than normal while you are getting used to the changes in the intake of carbs.

Blood Sugar Issues or Diabetes

Some people that try the keto diet will have problems with some low blood sugar or hypoglycemia at the beginning. This could be dangerous if you can't get your blood sugar stabilized while taking your diabetes medications.

There is evidence that shows diabetes can be prevented or slowed down with a healthy diet and exercise. To keep you safe, if you have a history of prediabetes, diabetes, or hypoglycemia, you shouldn't try the keto diet without talking to your doctor first.

With the changes to your diet and any weight might mean the dosage of your diabetes medication might need to be adjusted. You shouldn't follow any type of restrictive diet without being supervised by your doctor.

Other Medicines

Other medications shouldn't cause any major risks but might need to be looked at to make sure you are still in need of it. Your doctor will be able to tell you if any changes are needed.

Blood pressure medicines might need to be regulated by your doctor, since your blood pressure might go down while on a keto diet.

Nutrient Deficient or Underweight

Even though the keto diet is a high-fat diet, it could lead to weight loss and this might happen very quickly. If you are already underweight, have any mineral or vitamin deficiencies because you aren't eating enough, or have had any eating disorders in the past, you should not do this diet.

If you have a low BMI and want to try the keto diet to help improve your blood sugar level but aren't looking to lose weight, you absolutely must talk to your doctor or a dietitian before you start this diet. They can help you modify the diet to make sure your weight won't be affected.

If you can lose weight easily, a diet that includes complex carbs along with a lot of healthy fats and proteins might be a better fit for you.

If you have undergone gastric bypass surgery, this diet could be extremely dangerous for you since the risk of nutrient deficiencies might happen from not consuming enough calories.

Gall Bladder Removal or Gallstones

People that have had gallstones were told to stay away from fat but this isn't true now. The NHS says that low-fat diets could actually cause gallstones to grow.

If you have gallstones now, eating more fat might cause you some pain. If you want to try the keto diet, you may need to go very slow or try the diet after your gallstones have been removed or dissolved.

A study done in 2014 showed that high-fat diets might actually prevent gallstones from forming which may be a long-term benefit of the keto diet.

Even though the gallbladder has bile in it that helps to break down fats, it has been reported that by following a high-fat, low-carb diet without having a gallbladder can be successful.

Many people without gall bladders have been very successful on the keto diet without reporting any adverse side effects.

Kidney Stones or Kidney Disease

Kidney stones are a side effect that has been caused by the keto diet. If you have a history of kidney disease, it probably isn't worth the risk of trying the keto diet.

If you have a family history of any kind of kidney disease, you must talk with your doctor before beginning the keto diet. Your doctor will need to check your creatinine/calcium ratio to make sure you aren't risking any complications such as nephrolithiasis which is a dangerous level of calcium in the kidneys.

Children

The keto diet has been used for many years in children who have seizures to help keep them under control. This must be done under the supervision of a doctor.

There are some things to keep in mind before starting a keto diet to make sure all the macronutrients are balanced and appropriate for children.

You absolutely must consult your doctor or dietitian before beginning keto diet on any child.

Enzyme Deficiency or Defect

These disorders are extremely rare, but there are two serious contraindications of the keto diet called porphyria and pyruvate carboxylase deficiency. These conditions are caused by problems with the production of heme and lipid metabolism. Heme is found in hemoglobin that carries oxygen out of the lungs and into other parts of the body.

People that have these disorders will have deficiencies with certain enzymes that will make it hard to metabolize large amounts of free fatty acids. They will then transport them to the cell's mitochondria to create energy. If you are on the keto diet and have these deficiencies or other types of beta oxidations defects, it could cause extremely dangerous complications like mental changes, irregular heartbeats, and nervous system deterioration.

Free fatty acids get built up in the body and can't be used for energy. This is the main reason it is dangerous. People who have porphyria and pyruvate carboxylase deficiency need a steady supply of glucose to give their organs energy. If there isn't any glucose present due to the keto diet, some life-threatening problems might happen. This is called a catabolic crisis. To stay away from these complications, if you have a family history of mitochondrial disorders or suspect you might have any of these conditions, you must be tested by your doctor before you even think about going on the keto diet.

Exercise

Everyone knows that when you exercise, you are going to have better health. When you follow a keto diet, you are going to lose weight fast and improve your health. What would happen if you combined the two?

It would be reasonable to assume, if you combined the two it would take your weight loss and health to another level. The truth is a bit more complicated. With being restricted on your intake of carbs, there is a huge amount of change that is going to happen, and some of these are going to affect your exercise.

With the restrictive intake of carbs, you are limiting your muscle cells from getting glucose, which has always been the easiest fuel source. When our muscles can't access glucose, their high-intensity function is impaired. High intensity stands for any activity that lasts longer than ten seconds. The reason for this is that after ten seconds of maximum effort, the muscles begin turning to glucose for energy through a metabolic pathway known as glycolysis instead of the phosaphen system.

Fat and ketones aren't a good substitute for glucose during this time. Only after you have been exercising for two minutes will your body shift into this metabolic pathway that will use your fat and ketones.

Basically, when you restrict your intake of carbs, you deprive the cells in your muscles of glucose, which they need for fuel during the high-intensity effort for ten seconds to two minutes. This just means that if you are doing a ketogenic diet, it is going to limit your performance during exercises such as:

- Swimming or sprinting for more than ten seconds.

- Weightlifting for more than five reps each set using a weight that is heavy enough to bring you close to failure.

- High-intensity circuit training or interval training.

- Playing a sport that gives you minimal breaks like soccer, lacrosse, and rugby.

This list isn't a comprehensive one, but it gives you a good idea of the types of exercises that your body uses glycolysis for. Remember though, that the metabolic pathway timing all depends on each individual person. There are some that can maintain performance for 30 seconds without needing any carbs.

It is also important that you eat the right amount of proteins and fats when you are exercising while following a keto diet.

Many health professionals, when designing a diet plan, will set the protein intake first. Protein gets the top priority because it performs many actions that fats and carbs can't. Protein helps to make you feel fuller longer, has a better thermic effect, and stimulates muscle synthesis better than any other macronutrients. If you don't eat enough protein, you might wind up losing muscle mass and consuming more calories than you need.

If you are going to keep your exercise regimen or begin one, which you really should, you need to make sure you eat the correct amount of macros. Here are some guidelines to follow.

- The biggest part of excess calories should come from healthy fats, not from carbs or protein.
- Keep your protein intake to a gram per pound of body weight.

- Be sure that your caloric intake stays around a deficit of 250 to 500 calories. This isn't of top priority. Many people won't worry about calories that much when doing a keto diet.

Now that we've established that you need to be smart and careful when eating while exercising, let's take a closer look at some specifics.

Keto and Cardio

Luckily for the majority of us, we aren't athletes so adding in an exercise routine isn't going to be that hard. Cardio workouts don't require you to exercise at high-intensities which require your body to burn glycogen and sugar for results. You just have to bring your heart rate up and keep it there.

Because cardio has a low to moderate intensity, a keto diet isn't going to impair your performance. You might even realize that you can work out longer without getting as tired when you are in ketosis.

The intensity you need to aim to get the most out of your workout is moderate intensity. When you are aiming for moderate-intensity physical activity, you should get your heart rate to about 50 to 70 percent of your maximum heart rate.

In order to estimate your maximum heart rate, begin by subtracting your age from 220. If you are a 50-year-old person, to figure out your age-related heart rate, you would take 220 and subtract 50. This gives you a total of 170 beats per minute. Then you could figure out the 50 to 70 percent levels, which will be:

- 70 percent – 170 x 0.70 = 119
- 50 percent – 170 x 0.50 = 85

This means a 50-year-old person, in order to partake in moderate-intensity physical activity needs to keep a heart rate between 85 and 119 beats per minute.

While your body is adapting to a ketogenic diet, you need to try to aim for the bottom end of that range. When you have been on the diet for a couple of weeks, you will begin to realize you can maintain a higher heart rate without needing extra carbs.

If you are new to working out and cardio, you want to stick to 50 percent of your maximum heart rate for about 10 to 15 minutes. You can begin to increase the duration by 5 or so each week until you are able to work out for 30 to 45 minutes at 50 percent of your maximum heart rate. When you have managed this, you can begin increasing your intensity level every week until you've reached 70 percent of your maximum heart rate.

If you aren't sure what works best for cardio workouts, here are a few examples.

- Interval training classes
- Aerobic training classes
- Cycling
- Swimming
- Recreational sports
- Circuit training
- Running

You need to remember though, that your power and strength could end up being decreased in these workouts because of carb restriction. If you are aiming for a good cardiovascular workout, then it isn't important that you push yourself to the max for your power and strength.

This isn't saying you can't increase your power and strength while doing a keto diet. All you have to do to achieve this is practice some mindful exercising.

Weight Lifting and Keto

You can increase muscle mass, power, and strength while following a keto diet. The best thing is that you can improve all of these things at the same time by using the same program.

Remember that I stated earlier that without glucose your body can only last for ten seconds when doing high-intensity exercises? This means that if you are a weightlifter, you can improve your power and strength, as well as muscle mass by doing sets that don't last longer than ten seconds.

This means that if you follow a program that requires five or more sets of five or fewer reps for each of the exercises, then this is perfect for people on a keto diet.

Some recent research has found that lower reps can be helpful when it comes to hypertrophy. This means that your muscles don't need you to pump out 8 to 12 reps in a row to grow bigger. What the muscles are looking for is the right amount of volume, which all depends on the individual person, and for your volume to increase every week.

This means that you are able to build muscles without carbs. Carbs might be needed for some high-intensity work, but a bodybuilder does not have to consume lots of carbs in order to see results.

Supplementing

There are a lot of no carb supplements out there that can help boosts your exercise performance while following a keto workout. Here are some keto friendly supplements.

1. Creatine

This is one of the most well-studied exercise supplement and it is an effective and safe way to enhance the body's phosphagen system. This is why creatine is best for explosive weightlifter and athletes.

Consuming five grams each day of creatine monohydrate powder is a great way to supplement for people who are looking to increase their muscle mass, power, and strength.

2. MCT or Medium Chain Triglycerides

MCTs as stated earlier are a form of saturated fats that get sent straight to the liver once they have been digested. The liver uses these fats for more ketones and is then sent to the cells that need the energy. MCTs are a great option for endurance athletes and cardio training.

It is recommended that you supplement with one or two tablespoons of MCT oil or powder before doing any endurance workouts to get an extra boost of energy

3. Exogenous ketones

These ketones, much like ketone esters and ketone salts, can provide you with an instant source of energy. There is a downside though. This supplement might end up lowering your liver's production of ketones, so it would be best if you used these with MCTs to boost ketone production.

A lot like MCTs, exogenous ketones are great for endurance and cardio training athletes. The main thing is to be sure you stay well hydrated when using these supplements because they do have a diuretic effect.

4. Caffeine

It isn't surprising that caffeine has been discovered as a great way to improve exercise performance because of its stimulatory effects. However, you could end up finding that you no longer get the same boost when you begin taking caffeine on a constant basis because of the way the body adapts to the habitual intake.

Plus caffeine might end up increasing your cortisol levels, which end up decreasing your ketone production. It is best if you experiment with the other supplements and limit the amount of caffeine you use.

5. Taurine

This is an organic acid that has been found to help exercise performance. In fact, researchers have discovered that it works better to help exercise performance than caffeine.

In a recent study, the scientists looked at the effects that taurine, caffeine and taurine, and caffeine had on fatigue and power on all-out cycling sprints. The taurine supplement that was used by itself was able to decrease fatigue and improve power than the other two supplements.

This has a big implication for bodybuilders and athletes who follow a keto diet because this study looked at the energy system that tends to be the most affected by carb restriction. According to the study, the participants took 50 mg of taurine per kilogram of weight. This would probably be a safe metric to use to figure out how much you need to take. You can also slowly decrease the amount to see if you still get any effects.

6. Fish oil

The omega 3 fatty acids, EPA, and DHA found in fish oil help to boost your recovery and stimulate muscle synthesis. The AHA recommends that you consume one gram of these each day. This can be reached through a fish oil supplement or by eating three ounces of salmon or sardines each day.

The goal of this is to help reduce your soreness. That means you need to aim for a six-gram dose that is spread throughout the day.

7. Protein Powder

While it is best for you to consume the majority of your protein from natural sources, protein powder is a good idea when you need help meeting your protein needs. This is also great if you follow a vegan keto diet.

You should make sure that you stick with complete protein powders such as collagen, whey, casein, or a mix of plant proteins. Stay away from BCAA and EAA supplements because you will receive better benefits from a complete protein powder.

Use this by adding 20 to 40 grams of protein powder to a smoothie or you could consume it after you work out to help stimulate muscle synthesis without affecting your ketosis.

8. Beta-alanine

This is a common compound in more pre-workout supplements that will give your body a tingly sensation. Most people report that they are able to perform one or two reps more when they are training in sets of eight to 15 when they take beta-alanine.

This means that this is probably a really good supplement for keto dieters that need a better glycolytic pathway to help them through their training. High-intensity athletes and bodybuilders will get the most from this supplement.

With this supplement, timing doesn't really matter. Aim for two to five grams of beta-alanine along with five grams of creatine each day. If you don't enjoy the tingly sensation that it gives you, you can take a gram of beta-alanine two to five times during the day.

9. Alpha GPC

Choline is an important part of your nervous system. Whenever you move a muscle in your body, choline is needed in order to activate acetylcholine, a neurotransmitter which will send a chemical signal to your muscles and will make them mobile. The best way to get more choline is through taking an alpha GPC supplement.

Research has found that 600 mg of it can help to enhance your power output and your secretion of growth hormones. This suggests that this choline supplement is great for weightlifters and athletes.

10. L-citrulline

This is a common supplement for cardiovascular health supplement and sports performance. Some studies have discovered that supplements of L-citrulline help to improve endurance and reduce fatigue for anaerobic and aerobic prolonged exercise. This is a great supplement for nearly every active person, except for those who rely on the phosphagen system such as powerlifters and golfers. To help your exercise endurance, take 6,000 to 8,000 mg around an hour before you are going to work out.

Keto and Exercise in Harmony

To mix these two things, you have to make the right changes to your diet and workout program so that you don't cause any adverse reactions especially if you partake in high-intensity workouts.

When you are trying to add in exercise just to improve your health, then you can experiment with things a bit more than an athlete can. In general, you should try lifting weight and some cardio training every week. Cardio should be done two to three times each week and lift weights two to three times each week. You should avoid doing them both on the same day.

Keto While Vegan

Health, animal suffering, and climate change are three big issues that can be taken care of with a single solution, a vegan diet. At least, that's what a lot of health documentaries talk about. However, there is a more nuanced

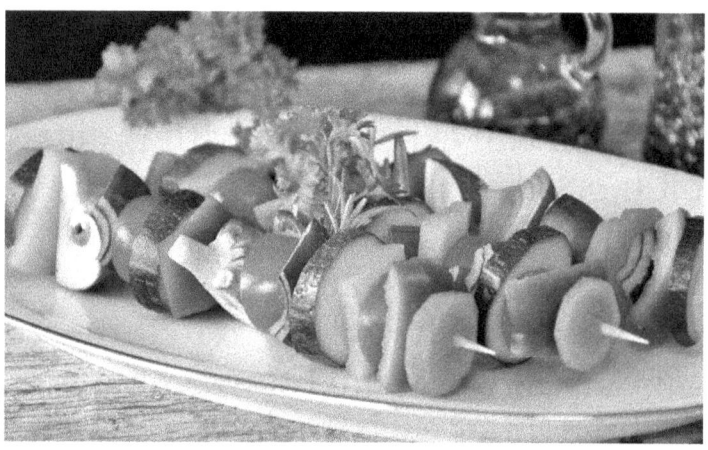

truth.

There are some that do better when they follow a low-carb diet with animal products, and then there are others that like a high-carb vegan diet. Following a vegan diet may not be the best diet for every health problem. For example, people that have epilepsy, Alzheimer's disease, Parkinson's disease, type 1 diabetes, type 2 diabetes, and obesity are helped tremendously when following a keto diet, while a vegan diet doesn't help them as much.

Now, does this mean that vegans need to give up their ethical concerns and start eating animal products? No. What should you do if you are following a high-carb vegan diet that isn't working for you and a keto diet could be exactly what you need, but it normally has too many animal products? Mix them.

An Overview

A vegan keto diet is an extremely restrictive diet, but you can pull it off and maintain your sanity, improve your health, and decrease animal suffering. In order to implement this correctly, follow these rules:

- Lower your carb intake to 35 grams or less.
- Get rid of all fish, meat, and other animal products.
- Consume plenty of veggies that are low in carbs.
- Make sure at least 70% of your calories are coming from plant-based fats.
- 25% of your calories need to come from plant-based proteins.
- Make sure you take supplements for your nutrients that you aren't getting from foods such as taurine, zinc, iron, EPA & DHA, B6, B12, and D3.

Limiting Carbs

It probably seems difficult enough to restrict the number of carbs you consume on a regular keto diet, so how is it going to go when you are following a vegan keto diet? Let's start out simply by looking at high-carb foods that you need to completely get rid of.

- Never Eat
    - Tubers like yams and potatoes.
    - Fruits like oranges, bananas, and apples.
    - Sugar like maple syrup, agave, and honey.
    - Legumes like peas, black beans, and lentils.
    - Grains like cereal, rice, corn, and wheat.

Now, the important part is finding vegan-friendly foods that are also low in carbs.

- Do Eat
    - Vegan protein like seitan, tofu, and tempeh.
    - Mushrooms like lion's mane, king oyster, and shiitake.
    - Leafy greens.
    - All above ground veggies like zucchini, cauliflower, and broccoli.
    - High-fat vegan dairy like vegan cheese, coconut cream, and coconut-based yogurt.

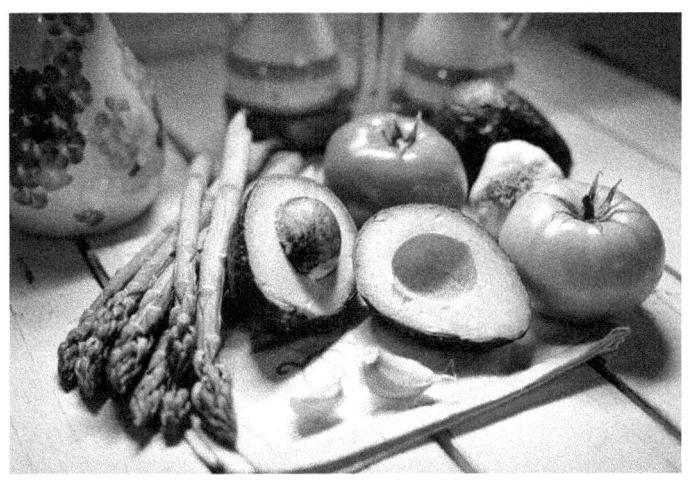

- Seeds and nuts like pumpkin seeds, sunflower seeds, almonds, and pistachios.
- Berries and avocado.
- Fermented foods like kimchi, sauerkraut, and natto.
- Sea vegetables like kelp, bladderwrack, dulse.
- Sweeteners like monk fruit, erythritol, and stevia.

- Other fats like avocado oil, MCT oil, olive oil, and coconut oil.

When you stick to the foods that are on the do eat list, you should be able to stick with a vegan keto diet and make sure that all of your nutritional bases are covered. At first though, you could find it difficult to adapt to this way of eating when many keto and low-carb recipes contain animal products. Luckily, all you have to do is make a couple of simple substitutions in order to veganize your keto recipes.

Simple Alternatives

If you buy a keto cookbook or search online for keto recipes, you are going to see a lot of recipes with cheese and eggs. There are also a lot of desserts full of high-fat dairy. That's where keto-friendly vegan substitutions come in.

- Substitute milk with coconut milk. The substitution works one to one, so if it calls for a cup of milk, use a cup of coconut milk.

- Substitute heavy cream with coconut cream. Depending on the creaminess of your coconut cream, you may find that you have to mix in some water or some of the water in the container.

- Replace butter with vegan butter or coconut oil. Coconut oil has a lower melting point but has the same smoke point as butter. This makes it a good replacement. If you don't like coconut oil, you can also use vegan butter. Check to make sure that there aren't any hydrogenated oils in the vegan butter because these increase your risk of heart disease.

- Instead of dairy cheese, use vegan cheese. There are a lot of vegan cheeses out there. If you don't want to use soy, then you can go for cashew, coconut, or other tree-nut cheeses.

- Replace cream cheese with vegan soft cheese. The company Treeline creates lots of cashew-based soft cheese and its texture is nearly identical to cream cheese. There are also ways to make your own cashew cheese.

- Instead of sour cream or yogurt, use nut-based yogurt. You can find coconut milk yogurts almost everywhere now and you may be able to find cashew or almond based yogurts. Check to make sure that there aren't any hidden sugars or carbs.

When you are purchasing keto-friendly vegan products, you need to check to make sure that they haven't added any sugars and that there aren't any hidden carbs or unhealthy ingredients such as hydrogenated oils. There are some products that use "gum" such as guar gum or agar agar. These are all compounds that are used to make them creamier and most people don't have a problem eating them. However, these products will cause gastrointestinal discomfort for some people, so check to see if your vegan dairy products have these added gums.

The great thing is that the availability of keto-friendly, dairy-free products have increased quickly. There are even some products that can be shipped straight to your home like Miyoko's Kitchen.

Now that we have looked at keto-friendly and vegan-friendly dairy choices, what to do about eggs? Eggs, egg yolks, and egg whites are important parts in a lot of delicious ketogenic recipes. As a vegan, do you need to ditch these?

Egg Substitutes

It can be so frustrating to find delicious but almost-vegan friendly recipes. You scroll through the list of ingredients and then you find it needs eggs. You don't have to fret just yet. You don't have to give up on these delicious foods. There are a lot of egg substitutes that you can use that are keto-friendly.

- Flax Seed

Ground up flax seeds makes a great binder. It tastes a bit nutty and works well in recipes that call for coconut or almond flour. Mix together a tablespoon of ground flax seeds with three tablespoons of water to replace an egg in a recipe.

- Silken Tofu

This is silkier and softer form of tofu that creates a great dairy and egg replacement. It's pretty much flavorless, but it may end up making your baked goods a bit dense, so it works best in brownies and some cakes and quick bread. A quarter of a cup of pureed silken tofu will replace an egg.

- Vinegar and baking soda

This is a good substitute for fluffier baked goods. A teaspoon of baking soda combined with a tablespoon of white vinegar will replace an egg.

If you don't want to make your own replacements, you can purchase ready-made vegan replacements.

- The Vegg

This company is 100% plant-based. They use only natural ingredients to create products that simulate the function, taste, and texture of eggs and it costs almost the same as real eggs.

- Follow Your Heart's VeganEgg

This is another plant-based company that makes vegan choices from mayo to cheese. That means they even have vegan eggs. Their VeganEgg is a whole egg replacement that has the texture and taste of actual eggs. These can be used to make cakes, muffins, and cookies. You can also scramble them up or use them to create omelets.

The main issue with these replacements is that they don't have the same protein or fat as a regular whole egg. This could make meeting all of your recommended macros on keto a little bit harder. Luckily, there are a lot of fats that you can eat from plant-based oils and lots of protein from vegan meat options.

Getting Enough Fat

While you aren't able to eat dairy, butter, meat, or eggs, you still have a lot of sources for fat on a vegan keto diet. Here are the best oils that you can have.

- Coconut oil

This is a great source of fat for baking, cooking, desserts, and fat bombs. It provides you with medium and long-chain saturated fatty acids that are a great source for fuel.

- Olive oil

This can be used to enhance the fat content and flavor a lot of dishes. Make sure that you keep temperatures under 405 degrees so that it doesn't end up oxidizing.

- Avocado oil

This oil has healthy monounsaturated fats than all of the other common oils. It also has the best smoke point at 520 degrees, which means it's great for deep frying, baking, and cooking.

- Red Palm oil

This is a great source of Vitamins A and E. It has a carrot-like flavor and buttery, rich texture. Its smoke point is a bit higher than coconut and olive oil. You do need to be careful when buying palm oil. There are a lot of palm oil products that are created in a way that hurts the wildlife, environment, and the workers that produce it.

That's why when you buy palm oil, look for bottles marked RSPO-certified or CSPO products. All of these companies produce products that are approved by the Roundtable on Sustainable Palm Oil. They use practices that meet strict social and environmental criteria. When you choose these products, you will be helping sustainable oil producers.

- MCT oil

This is often derived from palm and coconut oil. It is a medium chain triglyceride. These are saturated fatty acids that don't go through normal fat digestion and will head straight to your liver where it is changed into ketones. When you are looking for an energy boost, these can be added to hot drinks, fat bombs, sauces, and salads.

There are many other vegan oil options out there, but the ones listed provide you with health benefits and versatility. However, you aren't stuck with just oils to get your fat intake. You can find fat, as well as minerals and vitamins in these other foods: avocado, nuts, seeds, and vegan dairy substitutes.

With all of these fat-packed plant foods and oils, you shouldn't have a problem with getting the fats that you need on your vegan keto diet. The next thing you have to take care of, and probably the hardest, is getting your protein.

Vegan Protein Sources

Making sure that you get enough protein to maintain your health and muscle mass is hard enough for vegans, now you have to work with a keto diet. When you mix these diets, you are getting rid of a lot of amazing plant-based protein sources such as legumes.

When you can't have peas, lentils, and beans, how are you going to consume any protein?

Don't worry, there are other options.

- Tofu

This is a great substitute for all types of meats. Tofu is made from soybeans and contains lots of calcium and protein. While it does have a reputation of being blank, it has a great ability to absorb flavors from marinades and spices. If you make sure that you season your tofu before cooking it, it should taste delicious. You can also adjust the firmness and chewiness by purchasing extra-firm tofu and pressing out the water.

Since many vegan protein options contain soy, it's important to understand soy. Soy contains goitrogens, which can affect the thyroid. If you eat a lot of soy products and start experiencing unexplained weight gain, dry skin, constipation, cold sensitivity, and fatigue, you should limit your soy intake.

- Tempeh

This is a grainier and firmer tofu. This is made from fermented soybeans and is great to use for recipes calling for ground beef and fish. Tempeh doesn't have to be pressed like tofu, so only less step.

- Seitan

This is known as wheat meat and is made from seaweed, garlic, ginger, soy sauce, and wheat gluten. This is a great source of iron, low in fat and high in protein. If you are sensitive to gluten, you may want to avoid this protein source.

There are other "meat" sources that you can find in grocery stores. When you are trying to pick one out, make sure you read through the nutrition facts and ingredients. You don't want a product that has a lot of carbs or sugars. Try to find ones with the simplest ingredients and lowest carb content.

You can also turn to seeds and nuts to provide you with protein. They also contain important minerals and nutrients. Some good options are flaxseeds, sunflower seeds, almonds, pistachios, and pumpkin seeds. Make sure that you don't eat too many because they can rack up carbs.

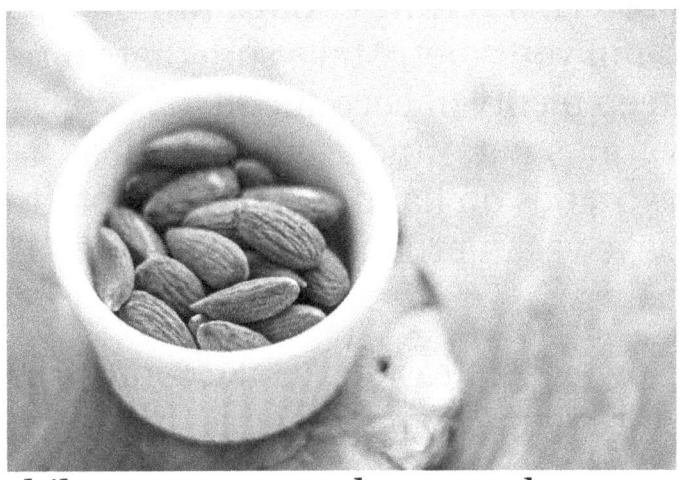

While peanuts are a legume, they are one of the only legumes that you can eat. They are low in carbs and high in protein.

The last vegan protein source is vegan protein powder. This is going to be your secret weapon. You can add flavorless vegan protein powders to your dishes to increase your protein content.

It is easier now to keep up with a vegan keto lifestyle. There are a lot of alternatives to dairy and eggs to help make veganizing your keto recipes easier. You shouldn't have any problems getting enough protein and fat in your diet. Make sure that you keep plenty of coconut oil, olive oil, various nuts, and seeds, as well as avocados on hand. Also, you should have vegan protein powder in your pantry.

Now, it's up to you to take control and start your vegan ketogenic diet.

FAQ

The majority of these questions have already been answered in the book but this section provides you with a quick reference guide to the most common questions that people have about the keto diet. If this doesn't give you enough in-depth answers, look for the chapter about your question.

Should I take supplements?

If you begin to feel a bit "crampy" or just don't feel like your normal self after you have begun a keto diet, you might want to look into certain supplements that will help you begin to feel better:

- Vitamin B Complex
- Multivitamins for Men
- Potassium Supplement
- Magnesium Supplement
- Vitamin D Supplement
- Multivitamins for Women

Always talk to your doctor before adding any supplements or vitamins to your diet.

Should I worry if I exercise?

There are usually two types of people that exercise. People that lift weights and people that run. If you do cardio exercises like running, biking, or participating in marathons, you really don't have to worry. Endurance training can be affected by the keto diet.

When lifting weights, you need to know what end results you want. Carbs could help your overall performance and help your muscles recover. By doing this, you will get better strength performance and faster gains when exercising. You can achieve this in a couple of ways, CKD and TKD.

CKD stands for the cyclical ketogenic diet and is a technique that is a bit more advanced. If you are just beginning keto, you don't need to do this. This is used more for competitors and bodybuilders. They used keto to help with building muscles while working out. To do this method, you do a normal keto diet for five days and then change to consuming more carbs for two days. By doing this, you will replenish all the glycogen stores in your body that will help you with the training that you do the other five days. Your goal is to get rid of all the stored glycogen.

TKD stands for the targeted ketogenic diet. With this technique, you eat carbs just before you workout to bump you out of ketosis when you exercise. It works by giving your muscles a needed supply of glycogen to use while working out. Once you have used up all this glycogen, your body will go back into ketosis.

My weight loss has stalled. What can I do?

Everybody on this planet who has ever attempted dieting has reached a weight loss plateau. There are a few things that might cause this to happen. There are many things that could help you over it. You could try fat fasting, intermittent fasting, change your eating habits, and cut out certain foods.

Here are some suggestions that might help you start losing weight again.

- Cut out processed foods
- Change to measuring yourself instead of weighing
- Stop consuming artificial sweeteners
- Lower the amount of carbs you consume
- Check all foods for hidden carbs
- Don't eat nuts
- Stop consuming dairy
- Increase your fat intake

What about alcohol?

You can drink alcohol while on a keto diet but you have to be careful. There are certain types of alcohol that do contain carbs.

If you absolutely have to drink, go for straight liquor. Don't drink cocktails, wine, or beer because these have carbs in them. Clear liquors are best. Just try to stay away from anything that is flavored. Those might have carbs in them.

I'm constipated. What can I do?

It is fairly normal for people who are just beginning the keto diet to start having irregular bowel movements. Here is a list of advice that can help with constipation or other bowel problems.

- o Try eating flax or chia seeds
- o Quit eating nuts (if you've been consuming a lot)
- o Try drinking hot tea or coffee

- Try eating a tablespoon of coconut oil
- Eat more veggies that are high in fiber
- Try a magnesium supplement
- Drink more water

I'm feeling very bad. What do I need to do?

The most common problems for anyone who has started the keto diet are getting brain fogginess and headaches. When our bodies go into ketosis, we start urinating a lot more than normal and we lose a lot of water. Along with that, our bodies are burning up the fat it has stored over the years. This easily leads to disaster. When you urinate, you are expelling a lot of electrolytes from your body and you have to replace them.

Try to eat more salt and drink more water. Salty foods like bacon, deli meat, and salted are good to eat while the body is transitioning to ketosis. Drinking bone broth will also help increase the electrolytes in your body. These will help keep you functional and sane.

What are macros and do I need to count them?

Macros stand for macronutrients. The main macronutrients are carbohydrates, proteins, and fats. As we stated earlier, calories do matter and you must keep track of them when on this lifestyle. It gets you in the habit of watching them. It also lets you see how well you are doing. It's amazing just how much we will lie to ourselves about the number of carbs we put into our diet.

Keeping track of your macros can also help you if your weight loss stalls. You can easily see the things in your diet that could be causing your problem. When you are tracking macros, be sure you use grams and not percentages. Many people who are new to this diet think that just because their diet consists of 75 percent fat, 20 percent protein, and 5 percent carbs, they are doing well. This might not be the case. Grams give you a more accurate description of what you have eaten.

If you get off some of your macros, it isn't a huge deal. There is some wiggle room to go up or down by 10 to 15 grams of proteins or fats the majority of the time. If you happen to go over sometimes, or under sometimes, don't beat yourself up too much. If you keep your calories under control and they aren't in a deficit too far, you are going to be fine.

Could I have a heart attack from eating too much fat?

The three groups of fat you will be consuming are monounsaturated fats, polyunsaturated fats, and saturated fats. People use to think that saturated fats were bad for you because of a link between heart disease and saturated fats. In recent years, it has been proven that saturated fats do NOT cause heart attacks but can actually improve your cholesterol levels. You can eat saturated fats without worrying.

Polyunsaturated fats are a bit trickier. Processed polyunsaturated fats like vegetable oils and margarine spreads are very bad for you. These are loaded with trans fats. These do have a connection with heart disease and you should stay away from them at all costs. There are some polyunsaturated fats that are natural in some foods like fish that can actually improve cholesterol. You should try to find as many of these healthy fats as you can and stop eating the unhealthy ones.

Monounsaturated fats are known as healthy ones. Olive oil is the main example of an oil that is more of a monounsaturated fat than anything else. It is very healthy for us and could help lower your cholesterol.

How does ketosis work?

Ketosis happens when you don't consume carbohydrates. When you don't eat carbs, your body will begin consuming your stored body fat for the energy it needs. It is extremely healthy for you and it is great for your brain.

How does your body get energy from fat? When your body goes into ketosis, it lets your lever break down fats into ketones. These ketones give us the energy we need.

 So, how does this add up to losing weight? When you have a caloric deficit, you aren't giving your body the energy it needs. Therefore, it has to dig into your stored fat to produce the energy it needs.

How to know if you are in ketosis?

Many people will use Ketostix to let them know when they get into ketosis. These can be found in most pharmacies. These are not very accurate. They generally let you know if you are or aren't in ketosis. If there is any purple or pink on the stick, this shows that your body is producing ketones. If the color is darker, it means you are dehydrated and your ketone levels are extremely concentrated.

Ketostix measures how much acetone is in the urine. These are also unused ketones. The ketone that your brain and body use for energy is called BHB or Beta-hydroxybutyrate. These are not measured by a Ketostix.

If you want results that are more accurate and reliable, you should use a blood ketone meter. These will show the correct amount of ketones that are in your blood. They don't get changed by hydration.

For more in-depth information, go back to the chapter on ketosis.

Will I lose a lot of weight?

The amount of weight you will lose is totally up to you. As stated earlier, exercising is going to cause you to lose more weight. If you can completely stop eating foods that cause weight loss stalls like dairy, artificial sweeteners, and wheat products. Wheat products are anything that has any identifiable wheat product, wheat flours, and wheat gluten in it.

Losing water weight is normal when beginning a keto diet. Getting into ketosis has a diuretic effect on your body that helps you lose a large amount of weight in just a couple of days. Remember, you won't be losing fat right now, just water. This shows that your body is starting to turn itself into a machine to burn fat.

Am I consuming too much fat?

Yes, you could eat too much fat. The main point is you need to be in a caloric deficit to be able to lose weight. If you consume too much fat, it is going to push you over this deficit and will cause you to go into surplus that will cause you to gain weight. Most people can't overeat when on the keto diet since it is very low in carbs but high in fats, it is entirely possible.

Find a keto calculator to help you calculate your macros so you can see how many carbs, proteins, and fats you have to eat every day. Remember when you do this, you change the number of carbs and proteins you need according to your activity level.

Do I have to count calories?

Yes, calories do matter. The number of calories you consume and work off is an easy equation but it will never be true for everybody. Food sensitivities, endocrine disorders, and metabolic disorders all play a part in this. So what should you do? Eat right. Don't ever go into the deficit with calories and don't eat foods that are on the bad list.

When doing a keto diet, you usually don't have to worry about calories since the proteins and fats fill you up and keep you feeling fuller longer. If you like exercising, you need to take care and make sure your calories don't get into the deficit. Make sure you eat enough to make up for what you lost when you exercised.

How do I track my intake of carbs?

The easiest way to keep track of your intake of carbs is by using MyFitnessPal with their mobile app. This app won't let you track net carbs but you can track the total carbs you eat along with your total fiber. You could get net carbs by subtracting your fiber intake from the total carb intake. There are other apps out there like FatSecret that helps track the carb intake. Just do some research and find one that works for you.

Where can I find recipes?

Almost any health-conscious website will have recipes for you to look at. You can always just Google what you are craving and you will be amazed at the number of recipes that will pop up. You can take your favorite recipe and convert them into low carb just by getting rid of the sugars and fruit in them. Instead of using sugar just substitute it for artificial sweeteners.

How quickly will I get into ketosis?

A keto diet isn't one that you can just pick and choose when you are going to do it. Your body has to adjust to the diet before it gets into ketosis and this will take time. This can take anywhere from two to seven days. It all depends on what you eat, your activity level, and your body type. The quickest way to get your body into ketosis is learning to exercise before you eat anything. Keep your carb intake to less than 20 grams each day. Remember to drink plenty of water.

Myths

The keto diet is all the rage now and you've probably heard a lot about it. You haven't tried it yet because you have heard all sorts of rumors. Let's talk about some of the most famous myths going around about the keto diet.

Everyone isn't going to get the keto flue and everyone's body is different and will react differently to this diet. Factors like your age, gender, overall health, and activity level will affect your metabolism, how healthy your hormones are, and how your body will adapt to ketosis. Let's look at these myths and find the truth behind them.

Keto is a high-protein, high-fat diet

The keto diet isn't like other low-carb diets or the Atkins Diet. It isn't high in protein. The intake of protein needs to be moderate because this helps your body get into ketosis and helps it say there. Eating too much protein is going to cause it to be changed into glucose. This won't help keep your glucose at low levels.

You are probably wondering just how much protein you need to consume. Normally, you need to get about 20 percent of your daily calories from protein, five percent needs to come from carbohydrates, and 75 percent will come from fat, where a low-carb, high-protein diet requires you to eat around 30 to 35 percent of your daily calories from protein.

You will just lose weight on this diet

This diet helps people lose weight and burn stored fat from their bodies. Even if you don't want to lose weight, you can still do this diet to maintain your weight. It can actually help you gain some weight.

Yes, you read that right. You can gain some weight while doing this diet. It is possible if you don't do it the correct way and your body doesn't get into ketosis.

There is a lot of controversy about diets that are low in carbs and high in fat because most people think you can only lose weight if you have a low-calorie intake. Others believe it is due to changes in the hormones that this diet causes. Most experts agree that the diet actually doesn't matter. If the calories you eat exceed the amount of activity you do, you are going to gain weight instead of losing it.

If you eat more calories than what your body needs, even if they are from healthy fats and protein, you are going to see an increase in the number on your scale.

If you don't want to lose weight, should you do this diet? There are numerous benefits of the keto diet that go beyond weight loss. This diet will help your body normalize blood sugar, improve digestive health, regulate hormone production, improve cognitive function, and could actually reduce the risk of getting heart disease or diabetes.

There's no science behind this diet

This is so false, it's hilarious. As stated earlier, this diet could help manage health problems such as Alzheimer's disease, cancer, epilepsy, muscle loss, high blood pressure, type 2 diabetes, dyslipidemia, obesity, and insulin resistance.

Can't exercise when doing keto

Exercising helps everybody, including people who are doing the keto diet. You may not feel energized when your body is transitioning into ketosis but this will lessen as your body adjusted to it. Even when you do high-intensity workouts, this diet won't cause any decline to your performance.

You don't have to stop working out when doing this diet. You may have to change up some of your workouts. If your body can handle it, exercising when you are in ketosis will help your body burn fat two to three times faster. This can help you maintain blood glucose levels. You might even notice you don't feel as fatigued.

To ensure you help your body while working out, make sure you eat enough calories especially those from fats. You need to let your body recover in between hard workouts.

If you are struggling while working out and you have a hard time recovering, try to eat more carbs right before you exercise. If you like to fast while doing the keto diet, save the high-intensity workout for when you have eaten more fuel.

You will lose muscle

This is another very false rumor. On the keto diet, you can actually gain muscle mass. If you can combine the keto diet with strength training, you could build muscle and increase your strength. The American Heart Association claims that these types of diets will cause a loss in muscle tissue. I don't know where they got that from but there are not any physiological requirements that humans have to eat carbs. This diet will not cause anyone to lose muscle mass.

Will this diet work if you don't exercise? Yes! It could lead to many improvements in your overall health. Exercising will kick things into high gear when talking about health benefits and body composition.

Everyone gets the keto flu

Every person is going to react differently to the keto diet. This makes it difficult to find out what side effects you are going to experience, how bad the effects are going to be, and how long they will last. Some people are going to transition into ketosis smoothly. Other may develop brain fog, sleep problems, more fatigue, and digestive problems for several weeks after getting into ketosis.

These side effects can be uncomfortable but they will go away in a week or so. You just have to be patient. You could lessen these by drinking more water, eating more fiber and salt, and getting more electrolytes from vegetables.

You won't have any energy doing keto

Many people say the energy and concentration increased after their body adjusted into ketosis. Your energy might be a bit lower when beginning this diet. After your body begins making ketones, it will give your brain a steady source of fuel. You might realize you are having better moods, the focus has increased, and you have more mental clarity after your body has become accustomed to the keto diet.

Remain on the diet for short periods of time

When you first begin the keto diet, you should just stay on this diet for two to three months and take a break. You have to give your body three weeks to get adjusted and then start back on the keto diet. If your body adjusts quickly to this, you can continue doing this for months and possibly years. Just listen to your body.

You can cheat on the keto diet

It really isn't realistic to remain on this diet for eternity. Cheat days are encouraged on other diets to give some support to your metabolism and to give you a break. When you cheat on the keto diet, it could bring you out of ketosis.

This may not be a problem if you do it intentionally. If you are aware of what is happening and can adjust your diet, coming out of ketosis is fine every now and then. If you realize you are no longer in ketosis since you have been cheating and consuming more carbs, take a few days to get back into eating right and cut back on the carbs.

You can eat any fat on keto just like with Atkins

Yes. Most of the calories on this diet come from fat. This isn't giving you permission to consume every saturated fat out there. Because keto isn't about just losing weight, you can eat healthy fats. Atkins lets you eat any fatty foods. Most people who try the keto diet want you to stay away from processed meats like bacon, salami, and sausage.

You are able to eat clean and avoid cheeses, poor quality meats, fried foods, processed foods, fast food, and trans fats if you want to get the most out of this diet. If you want to eat healthier, choose cage-free, organic eggs, pasture raised poultry, wild caught fish, avocados, nuts, grass-fed butter, grass-fed meats, and cold pressed oils like extra virgin olive oil or coconut oil.

Women and men are exactly the same with keto

Women are normally a bit more sensitive to dietary changes and weight loss than men. It might be possible for women to follow this diet and stay safe. They could also incorporate intermittent fasting if wanted. Women have to be sure they consume more non-starchy veggies to replenish their electrolytes and nutrients.

Women need to try to reduce the amount of stress that is in their lives and listen to their bodies. Stress can cause hormonal changes that can keep them out of ketosis. Pay attention to what your body is telling you when you workout. Exercise will impact your mood, your energy, how well you sleep, how much alcohol and caffeine you consume, how long you are out in the sun, and how many environmental toxins you are exposed to. If you start feeling run down or overwhelmed, you have to adjust your diet accordingly. If you push your body too hard, it might fight back.

You have to fast when doing keto

Fasting while on the keto diet isn't a requirement. You can choose whether or not you want to fast. You shouldn't fast until your body has adjusted into ketosis. After your body is used to consuming lower cabs, introducing intermittent fasting might have several benefits for your body. It could help with cravings, controlling hunger, speeding up weight loss, and detoxifying your body.

Some think that fasting is hard since you will feel hungry but this isn't true. If you eat the right amounts of veggies, protein, and fats, you are going to feel fuller longer. Fasting isn't as challenging as most people think it is.

No alcohol

Cocktails, beer, and wine are full of carbs. If you must have alcohol, there are options for you while doing the keto diet. Many liquors, light beers, and dry wines are very low in carbs.

You don't have to totally give up alcohol. You just need to be more conscious of what you are choosing. You need to also be careful when drinking because your body isn't full of carbs that absorb the alcohol. You might not be as tolerable to alcohol as you used to be. If you do drink, make sure you drink while you are eating since the fat and protein helps your body absorb the alcohol and prevents surges in blood sugar.

It's dangerous

Just like any diet or lifestyle change, there will be downsides but this diet isn't dangerous.

There are potential problems such as increased cholesterol and heart disease, gastrointestinal distress, decreased bone density, mineral and vitamin deficiencies, and kidney stones. These can be helped and avoided by adding supplements to your diet.

You absolutely have to keep yourself hydrated and go slowly into fasting if you have decided to. Be sure you know what your daily macros need to be and be sure you are hitting them. If you do all this, you will probably avoid all these problems.

Final thoughts

In spite of everything you have probably heard about the keto diet, it is relatively safe for most people to do for a long time. It could help you build muscles if you add in strength training. You might increase your energy levels due to your body burning more fat.

Most people think you only lose weight when doing the keto diet. The keto diet creates low energy and many other problems. Many think it is not safe for women to do for any amount of time since it could cause loss of muscle mass.

The keto diet is low in carbs and high in fats that will change the way the body burns fat for energy. It will stop burning sugar and carbs we eat and begin burning the fat that is stored in the body.

Good Foods

Now that you have all the information about the keto diet, let's find out exactly what you will be able to eat while on this new lifestyle. You will also get a list of what foods you need to avoid.

What to Eat

- Meats – all meats that are unprocessed are low in carbs and great for your new lifestyle. The

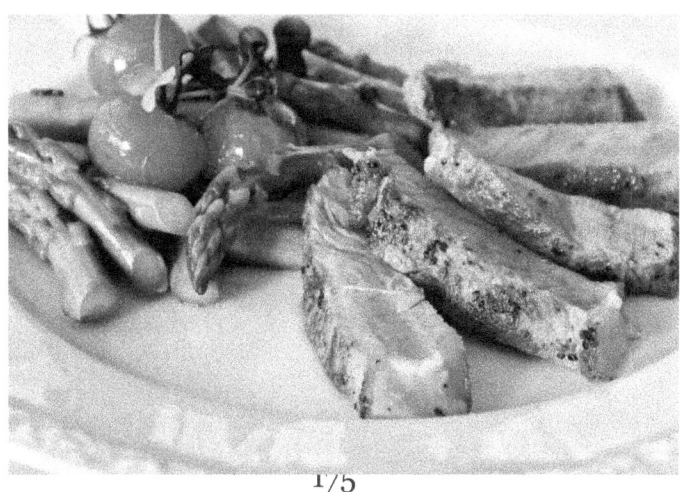

best for you are ones that are organic, grass-fed meats. You need to remember that you are eating more fats than protein, so don't go crazy with meats. Look out for processed meats such as sausages, cold cuts, and meatballs. They will sometimes contain added carbs.

- Seafood and fish – all fish are good options, especially salmon. Salmon is high in Omega 3 fatty acids which our bodies need.

- Eggs – these are the most versatile foods you can eat on this diet because they can be fixed in so many different ways.

- High-fat sauces – most of the fats you consume needs to come from sources such as meat, fish, and eggs. You can also use butter and coconut oil to cook with to add fats into your diet.

- Vegetables that grow above ground – choose vegetables that grow above ground like green vegetables. The best ones are:
    - Zucchini
    - Avocado
    - Kale
    - Cauliflower
    - Brussels sprouts
    - Cabbage
    - Green beans
    - Broccoli
    - Asparagus
    - Spinach
- Dairy that is high in fat – the more fat it has in it, the better it is for this diet. Butter is the best. Make sure to get real butter and not margarine. Cheese that is high in fat is also great. High-fat

yogurts need to be eaten in moderation. Normal milk is high in sugars so you need to stay away from it.

- Nuts – you can eat these in moderation. The best ones are Brazil, macadamia, and pecans.

- Berries – these can also be eaten in moderation. These include strawberries, blackberries, raspberries, and blueberries.

- Water – you absolutely have to drink a lot of water.

- Coffee – this is fine as long as you don't add anything to it except coconut oil and butter.

- Tea – this is also fine as long as you don't add sugar to it.

- Bone broth – consuming this can help add nutrients and electrolytes back into the diet.

- Alcohol – if you absolutely have to drink any alcohol, you can drink brandy, whiskey, vodka, and dry wine. Just make sure you don't consume anything that has added sugar.

- Dark chocolate – you need to find chocolate that has more

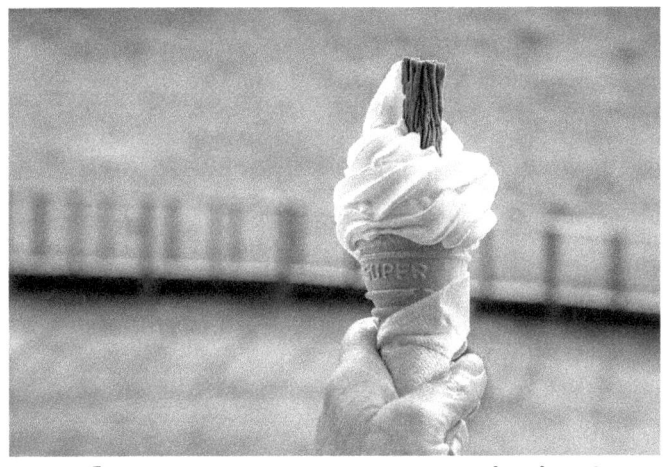

than 70 percent cocoa in it. 85 percent is the ideal amount.

Foods to Avoid

- Sugar – this is a huge no-no. You absolutely have to stay away from soft drinks, fruit juices, vitamin water, and sports drinks. You also have to stay away from these:
    - Donuts
    - Breakfast cereals
    - Sweets
    - Frozen treats
    - Candy
    - Chocolate bars
    - Cakes
    - Cookies
- Starches
    - Sweet potatoes
    - Porridge
    - Muesli
    - Bread

- Rice
- Potato chips
- Pasta
- French fries
- Beans
- Potatoes
- Lentils

- Beer – this is nothing more than liquid bread.
- Fruits
- Pre-packaged low-carb foods – these are not necessarily good for you. Be sure to read the label before you purchase these. Most of the Atkins products are not really low in carbs.
- Margarine – you have to use real butter. Never ever eat margarine, it is so bad for you.

Shopping List

In order to get you started on this diet the right way, this chapter is going to give you a shopping list that will help you get everything you are going to need. It has been organized by the types of food in order to help with your travels in the grocery store.

- **Vegetables**
  - Zucchini
  - Summer squash
  - Spaghetti squash
  - Sprouts
  - Garlic
  - Onions
  - Lettuce
  - Cucumbers
  - Bell pepper

- o Cabbage
- o Cauliflower
- o Broccoli

- **Fruits**
  - o Strawberries
  - o Raspberries
  - o Blackberries
  - o Blueberries
  - o Avocados

- **Seafood**
  - o Trout
  - o Tuna
  - o Shrimp
  - o Salmon

- **Meats**
  - o Pepperoni

- Luncheon meats – make sure you read the label to see if they have added nitrites or carbs
- Hotdogs
- Bratwurst
- Elk
- Buffalo
- Venison
- Ground lamb
- Lamb Chops
- Pork steaks
- Ham steaks
- Ground Pork
- Pork ribs
- Polish sausage
- Kielbasa
- Bacon

- Breakfast sausage
- Duck
- Whole chicken
- Chicken breast
- Chicken thighs
- Ribeye steak
- Chuck roast
- Ground beef 80/20
- **Dairy**
  - Greek yogurt
  - Hard cheeses
  - Butter
  - Sour cream
  - Eggs
  - Cream cheese
  - Heavy cream
- **Fats and oils**

- Sesame oil
  - Coconut oil
  - Grapeseed oil
  - Olive oil
  - Avocado oil
- **Miscellaneous**
  - Pork rinds
  - Olives
  - Beef jerky
  - Full-fat ranch dressing
  - Sugar-free salad dressings
  - Salsa
  - Hot sauce
  - Cider vinegar
  - Mustard
  - Pickle juice
  - Sugar-free pickles

- Chicken stock
- No-sugar-added sauces
- Nut Flours
- Seeds
- Nuts
- Almond butter
- Sunflower butter
- Peanut butter

30-Day Meal Plan

So that you can get started, here is your 30-day meal plan. Before you start, make sure that you know all of your macro numbers.

Day 1

Breakfast: Two eggs and two slices of bacon – 1 gram net carb

Lunch: An avocado with pork rinds – 2 grams net carb

Dinner: Tuna salad with two hard boiled eggs, bibb lettuce, a half cup of almonds, an apple, and a cucumber – 13 grams net carb

Day 2

Breakfast: Bulletproof coffee – 0-gram net carb

Lunch: Serving of sunflower seeds – 4 grams net carbs

Dinner: Two ounces of turkey breast, hard-boiled egg, a quarter cup of cherry tomatoes, an ounce of sharp cheddar, four pita bites, two tablespoons almonds – 13 grams net carbs

Day 3

Breakfast: One boiled egg with a tablespoon mayo – 1 gram net carb

Lunch: 1/3 cup of hummus with pork rinds – 9 grams of net carb

Dinner: Chicken salad with balsamic vinegar dressing – 6 grams net carb

Day 4

Breakfast: Romaine lettuce leaf with a half ounce of butter, an ounce of cheese, half avocado, and a cherry tomato – 3 grams net carb

Lunch: String cheese – 1 gram of net carb

Dinner: Two ounces of turkey breast, hard-boiled egg, a quarter cup of cherry tomatoes, an ounce of sharp cheddar, four pita bites, two tablespoons almonds – 13 grams net carbs

Day 5

Breakfast: Two scrambled eggs – 1 gram net carb

Lunch: 1/3 cup of hummus with pork rinds – 9 grams of net carb

Dinner: Chicken salad with balsamic vinegar dressing – 6 grams net carb

Day 6

Breakfast: Two scrambled eggs with an avocado and two ounces of smoked salmon – 5 grams net carb

Lunch: Full-fat laughing cow cheese – 1 gram net carb

Dinner: Tuna salad with two hard boiled eggs, bibb lettuce, a half cup of almonds, an apple, and a cucumber – 13 grams net carb

Day 7

Breakfast: Two fried eggs – 1 gram net carb

Lunch: 1/3 cup of hummus with pork rinds – 9 grams of net carb

Dinner: Chicken salad with balsamic vinegar dressing – 6 grams net carb

Day 8

Breakfast: Two hardboiled eggs mashed into three ounces of butter – 1 gram net carb

Lunch: Quest bar – 5 grams net carb

Dinner: Two ounces of turkey breast, hard-boiled egg, a quarter cup of cherry tomatoes, an ounce of sharp cheddar, four pita bites, two tablespoons almonds – 13 grams net carbs

Day 9

Breakfast: An avocado with three ounces of deli turkey, an ounce of lettuce, and an ounce and a half of cream cheese – 9 grams net carb

Lunch: Serving of pork rinds – 0 grams net carb

Dinner: Chicken salad with balsamic vinegar dressing – 6 grams net carb

Day 10

Breakfast: An avocado fill with a third of a cup of mayo and three ounces of smoked salmon – 6 grams net carb

Lunch: Full-fat laughing cow cheese – 1 gram net carb

Dinner: Roll three slices of cheese in three slices of turkey and serve with a half of an avocado, cucumber slices, blueberries, and almonds – 13 grams net carb

Day 11

Breakfast: A cup of coffee with four tablespoons heavy cream – 2 grams net carb

Lunch: An avocado with pork rinds – 2 grams net carb

Dinner: Tuna salad with two hardboiled eggs, bibb lettuce, a half cup of almonds, an apple, and a cucumber – 13 grams net carb

Day 12

Breakfast: Two eggs and two slices of bacon – 1 gram net carb

Lunch: Quest bar – 5 grams net carb

Dinner: Two ounces of turkey breast, hard-boiled egg, a quarter cup of cherry tomatoes, an ounce of sharp cheddar, four pita bites, two tablespoons almonds – 13 grams net carbs

Day 13

Breakfast: Two fried eggs – 1 gram net carb

Lunch: 1/3 cup of hummus with pork rinds – 9 grams of net carb

Dinner: Chicken salad with balsamic vinegar dressing – 6 grams net carb

Day 14

Breakfast: Two hardboiled eggs mashed into three ounces of butter – 1 gram net carb

Lunch: An avocado with pork rinds – 2 grams net carb

Dinner: Tuna salad with two hardboiled eggs, bibb lettuce, a half cup of almonds, an apple, and a cucumber – 13 grams net carb

Day 15

Breakfast: Bulletproof coffee – 0-gram net carb

Lunch: Serving of sunflower seeds – 4 grams net carbs

Dinner: Two ounces of turkey breast, hardboiled egg, a quarter cup of cherry tomatoes, an ounce of sharp cheddar, four pita bites, two tablespoons almonds – 13 grams net carbs

Day 16

Breakfast: An avocado with three ounces of deli turkey, an ounce of lettuce, and an ounce and a half of cream cheese – 9 grams net carb

Lunch: Serving of pork rinds – 0 grams net carb

Dinner: Roll three slices of cheese in three slices of turkey and serve with a half avocado, cucumber slices, blueberries, and almonds – 13 grams net carb

Day 17

Breakfast: One boiled egg with a tablespoon mayo – 1 gram net carb

Lunch: 1/3 cup of hummus with pork rinds – 9 grams of net carb

Dinner: Chicken salad with balsamic vinegar dressing – 6 grams net carb

Day 18

Breakfast: A cup of coffee with four tablespoons of heavy cream – 2 grams net carb

Lunch: An avocado with pork rinds – 2 grams net carb

Dinner: Tuna salad with two hard boiled eggs, bibb lettuce, a half cup of almonds, an apple, and a cucumber – 13 grams net carb

Day 19

Breakfast: Romaine lettuce leaf with a half ounce of butter, an ounce of cheese, half avocado, and a cherry tomato – 3 grams net carb

Lunch: String cheese – 1 gram of net carb

Dinner: Two ounces of turkey breast, hard-boiled egg, a quarter cup of cherry tomatoes, an ounce of sharp cheddar, four pita bites, two tablespoons almonds – 13 grams net carbs

Day 20

Breakfast: Two scrambled eggs – 1 gram net carb

Lunch: 1/3 cup of hummus with pork rinds – 9 grams of net carb

Dinner: Chicken salad with balsamic vinegar dressing – 6 grams net carb

Day 21

Breakfast: An avocado fill with a third of a cup of mayo and three ounces of smoked salmon – 6 grams net carb

Lunch: Full-fat laughing cow cheese – 1 gram net carb

Dinner: Roll three slices of cheese in three slices of turkey and serve with a half avocado, cucumber slices, blueberries, and almonds – 13 grams net carb

Day 22

Breakfast: An avocado with three ounces of deli turkey, an ounce of lettuce, and an ounce and a half of cream cheese – 9 grams net carb

Lunch: Serving of pork rinds – 0 grams net carb

Dinner: Chicken salad with balsamic vinegar dressing – 6 grams net carb

Day 23

Breakfast: Two hard boiled eggs mashed into three ounces of butter – 1 gram net carb

Lunch: Quest bar – 5 grams net carb

Dinner: Roll three slices of cheese in three slices of turkey and serve with a half avocado, cucumber slices, blueberries, and almonds – 13 grams net carb

Day 24

Breakfast: A cup of coffee with four tablespoons of heavy cream – 2 grams net carb

Lunch: An avocado with pork rinds – 2 grams net carb

Dinner: Two ounces of turkey breast, hard-boiled egg, a quarter cup of cherry tomatoes, an ounce of sharp cheddar, four pita bites, two tablespoons almonds – 13 grams net carbs

Day 25

Breakfast: Two fried eggs – 1 gram net carb

Lunch: 1/3 cup of hummus with pork rinds – 9 grams of net carb

Dinner: Chicken salad with balsamic vinegar dressing – 6 grams net carb

Day 26

Breakfast: Two eggs and two slices of bacon – 1 gram net carb

Lunch: An avocado with pork rinds – 2 grams net carb

Dinner: Tuna salad with two hard boiled eggs, bibb lettuce, a half cup of almonds, an apple, and a cucumber – 13 grams net carb

Day 27

Breakfast: An avocado with three ounces of deli turkey, an ounce of lettuce, and an ounce and a half of cream cheese – 9 grams net carb

Lunch: Serving of pork rinds – 0 grams net carb

Dinner: Chicken salad with balsamic vinegar dressing – 6 grams net carb

Day 28

Breakfast: Romaine lettuce leaf with a half ounce of butter, an ounce of cheese, half avocado, and a cherry tomato – 3 grams net carb

Lunch: String cheese – 1 gram of net carb

Dinner: Tuna salad with two hard boiled eggs, bibb lettuce, a half cup of almonds, an apple, and a cucumber – 13 grams net carb

Day 29

Breakfast: Bulletproof coffee – 0-gram net carb

Lunch: Serving of sunflower seeds – 4 grams net carbs

Dinner: Two ounces of turkey breast, hard-boiled egg, a quarter cup of cherry tomatoes, an ounce of sharp cheddar, four pita bites, two tablespoons almonds – 13 grams net carbs

Day 30

Breakfast: Two fried eggs – 1 gram net carb

Lunch: 1/3 cup of hummus with pork rinds – 9 grams of net carb

Dinner: Chicken salad with balsamic vinegar dressing – 6 grams net carb

Conclusion

Thank you for making it through the end of *The Ketogenic Diet for Beginners*. Let's hope it was informative and able to provide you with all of the tools you need to achieve your goals whatever they may be.

Losing weight has always been a struggle, but with the keto diet, it becomes easier. Use the information found in this book to help get you started on a ketogenic diet.

Finally, if you found this book useful in any way, a review on Amazon is always appreciated!

www.ingramcontent.com/pod-product-compliance
Lightning Source LLC
Chambersburg PA
CBHW051544020426
42333CB00016B/2085